REDIRECTING BOARDS:

A New Vision of Governance for Planned Parenthood

by R. James LeFevre

Published by Planned Parenthood Federation of America, Inc.
810 Seventh Avenue, New York, New York 10019

The views expressed in this book are those of the author and are not in their entirety necessarily held by Planned Parenthood Federation of America (PPFA) or its affiliates. The book was originally sponsored by PPFA. PPFA has registered the copyright and is responsible for marketing and distribution. Planned Parenthood of Northern New England (PPNNE) is an additional sponsor and it coordinated all aspects of the book's production.

Design by Eugenie S. Delaney
Typesetting by Fletcher Typesetting
Printed by Thomson-Shore, Inc.

Library of Congress Cataloging-in-Publication Data
LeFevre, R. James, 1944-
Redirecting boards : a new vision of governance for Planned Parenthood / by R. James LeFevre
p. cm.
Includes bibliographical references.
ISBN 0-934586-73-X
1. Planned Parenthood Federation of America—Management.
I. Planned Parenthood Federation of America. II. Title.
HQ766.5.U5L42 1993
363.9'6'06073—dc20 92-46519
CIP

TABLE OF CONTENTS

FOREWORD

Susan B. Anthony's admonition sounds just like the kind of fiery rhetoric that Margaret Sanger used as she lit the flames of the birth control movement at the beginning of this century.

For many of us involved with Planned Parenthood, Margaret Sanger would be the perfect volunteer leader for an affiliate's board of directors in this last decade of the twentieth century. Most likely, she would become chair after paying her dues by serving a successful obligatory stint as head of the bylaws committee. She would lead her board by rocking the boat, fighting the good fight for reproductive freedom, and dispatching her nominating committee to search for members of the board who would be risk takers and true believers. Ms. Sanger would know that it is the job of every Planned Parenthood affiliate board of directors to be the unwavering champion of reproductive freedom for all, that it is an enormous job, and that it is the continuation of over 75 years of revolutionary social change and justice. She would not be surprised to find that, because our mission is so fundamentally important, we are outspoken on its behalf and are sometimes seen as unpopular and uncompromising. She'd understand that Planned Parenthood boards must be able to take the heat and find the light. They must be prudent, yet not so cautious that they forget how to be daring when appropriate, and provocative when necessary.

"Cautious, careful people, always casting about to preserve their reputation and social standing, never can bring about reform.

Those who are really in earnest must be willing to be anything or nothing in the world's estimation, and publicly and privately in season and out, avow their sympathies with despised and persecuted ideas and their advocates, and bear the consequences."

SUSAN B. ANTHONY

They must be prepared to weather the storm of accusations, half-truths, and illegal attacks from the shrill minority (political bullies and terrorists) who attempt to shut them down.

> ***"Planned Parenthood is not just a national network of agencies; we're a movement. We don't primarily provide social services; we're out to change the world and rid it of the root causes of poverty and despair."***
>
> **ANNE SAUNIER**
> **Former Chair of the National Board**
> **Planned Parenthood Federation of America**

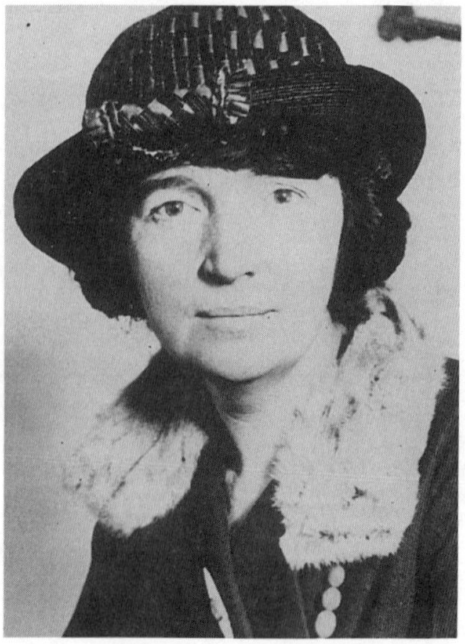

"Life has taught me we must put our convictions into action."

MARGARET SANGER
Founder, Planned Parenthood Federation of America

What I'm not sure about is whether Ms. Sanger would relish the meticulous revising of the annual budget line-items, coping with the regulations of the local United Way, or attending a board meeting in which most of the time was spent regurgitating the minutes of twelve different committees. At some point in the midst of all that, I can imagine her scrambling to her feet and yelling out a famous Ruth Green quotation, "But let's get on with it!"* It is this exasperated impatience to get on with the truly essential and to quit meddling in routine operations that would place Sanger squarely in the camp of organizational radicals ready to redefine and revamp what boards should do.

I don't mean to disparage the importance of traditional board activities and duties, such as serving on committees, overseeing budgets, and complying with local funding rules. Yet such activities, useful though they are, can also consume inordinate amounts of time and distract boards from other truly critical business. A successful board affirmatively chooses the right roles and tasks for itself and, as importantly, reduces the time spent on less important tasks, and altogether abandons those activities that are not in its province. Boards cannot do everything; there isn't enough time or energy. They must eliminate many of the activities that historically have preoccupied them so they can recapture adequate time to perform those unique functions that only boards can do.

---

* Ruth Green was the long-time executive director for Planned Parenthood in Tucson, Arizona. Her leadership and eternal impatience have been recognized in honoring her memory with the annual award named in her honor and presented at PPFA's Annual Meeting. This award goes to the executive director best exemplifying the ability to forge a board partnership in order for affiliates to have boards successful in public affairs, fund raising, and strategic planning.

Keeping up with Change. Nonprofit organizations, in response to a changing environment, have become very complicated and demanding. Furthermore, boards of directors are in need of dramatic re-examination because it is precisely in the board domain—the domain of vision, values, advocacy, fund raising—that the currents of change have affected Planned Parenthood so profoundly in this past decade. Management systems and philosophies have undergone massive changes. But have boards changed sufficiently to keep up with changing times? In many cases, the answer is no. Many are structured much as they were in the 1970s, operating in a business-as-usual straight jacket. An affiliate whose board is not operating with realistic and contemporary approaches has a fatal flaw.

The reality is that nonprofit boards of directors must reinvent the way they do business, refocus their roles to make their work manageable, and rid themselves of time-wasting activities. Even as they reform their more routine responsibilities, boards must keep Planned Parenthood affiliates lively, entrepreneurial, vibrant, and courageous. The Planned Parenthood movement must create a legacy of empowered affiliates providing powerful programs. Enlightened board governance is the vehicle that can get this done.

The board is the backbone of any affiliate's long-term success. Almost everyone interviewed for this book and every expert source agrees that *the single most important factor in the success of any nonprofit organization is the performance of the governing board.* Paul Hood, who has written much about nonprofit boards, suggests that an effective board "will attract a superior chief executive director who, in turn, will attract a highly capable and dedicated staff. The combination of these elements will attract important patronage and support to the organization. Thus, the successful nonprofit organization is composed of a series of building blocks with an effective governing board as the keystone."

The Future and the Job Undone. Many of us in the Planned Parenthood movement have a sense that we are poised on the threshold of an exhilarating new era. For example, *Planned Parenthood 2000* (the planning and discussion paper developed by the Metropolitan Executive Directors Council in 1987) optimistically suggests a future that makes our movement bigger, better, and stronger than we have ever been before. This blueprint document paints a picture of opportunity seized, threat vanquished, programs expanded, and finances developed. In fact, the image portrayed is a Planned Parenthood organization that has grown into a central and ubiquitous force in American life. But this optimistic notion for the future is almost totally dependent upon strong individual affiliates, capable of creating new and better answers to increasingly complex questions. Furthermore, our optimism has been challenged by the battle over the "gag rule" imposed by recent administrations, the Supreme Court decision in *Planned Parenthood v. Casey,* and other similar developments. The ability to survive—to preserve basic reproductive freedoms—may be the fundamental question. Given such issues, it is imperative for Planned Parenthood to have strong affiliates that can withstand attack. Wise governance is an important source of such institutional strength.

> ***"Nowhere is the principle of choice demonstrated so clearly as in our philanthropic organizations—where people freely choose to devote their own time, talents and resources to enhancing the quality of our lives . . ."***
>
> **JAMES GREGORY LORD**
> **Organization and Fund-raising Consultant**

We have a powerful sense of mission and conviction that the Planned Parenthood cause is part of the cutting edge for a fairer world and for global salvation. The realization that our work is not finished keeps us eager for even greater success. Jane Johnson, PPFA's Vice President for Affiliate Development and Education, makes the point that, "In the biographies of the healthy affiliate, one will almost always find people for whom no cause is more important. They are convinced that no perfect world could even be imagined until children have a reasonable chance of being born into a welcoming and nurturing environment. They surely understood that when women have no control over their childbearing, legions of undernurtured children and defeated, devastated women are the inevitable consequence. This scenario and prospect has never made sense to those who embrace the Planned Parenthood mission." (*The Mission Is The Message,* 1987.)

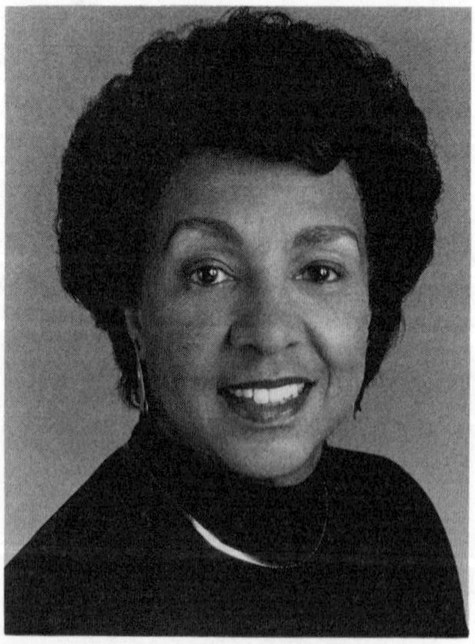

JANE JOHNSON
Vice President for Affiliate Development and Education
Planned Parenthood Federation of America

According to Roth Schleck, "it is our boards who are primarily the keepers of the faith, the stewards of the mission, the linkage to the broader community, the insurance policy for longevity and the trustee for the future." If our boards flounder, we are doomed to fail. As a federation, we must continue to examine the difficulties of governance, to understand what works and what doesn't, and to design a better structure and process for our boards, so that they will survive and thrive in the tumult of this decade. If we manage all this, we will have surely paid attention to the words of Susan B. Anthony to abandon our cautious ways; we will have paid tribute to the pioneering efforts and goals of Margaret Sanger. And the dreams of *Planned Parenthood 2000* will match their promises with deeds. "The role of the board," says Kenneth Dayton, "is to institutionalize the concept, the genius that created [the organization] . . ." The task of a Planned Parenthood board is to preserve the common sense and passion of small groups of community volunteers, meeting in kitchens and church basements, who worked and laughed, argued and planned, and who formed steering committees that ultimately led to the affiliates that we now serve.

A New Vision of Governance. My research and experience have led me to some very good news: Many Planned Parenthood boards are succeeding, are brimming with passion, and are raising more money than they ever have done before. *Planned Parenthood boards have not allowed themselves to be overwhelmed or crushed by the difficulties of board accomplishment.* In fact, they are often the very best board in a given community. Paradoxically, the reason our boards are in good shape is because of the very same thing that has almost driven us crazy: We have been under constant attack, and if our boards hadn't protected our mission from defeat, we would not have survived the last decade.

Yet there is more to be done. Even if affiliate boards are usually among the strongest, we can always get better. Even if affiliate performance is growing and expanding, boards can usually work smarter, if not harder. In fact, if Planned Parenthood boards are doing well, they must take the responsibility of continuing to evolve so they can be a shining light for other boards to look for.

The problem is not that our boards are broken. In virtually every case, we simply need to strengthen them, clarify their roles, give them better tools with which to do their work, free them from the unnecessary, and recruit and retain individuals whose talent lies in governance. At the same time, we can assist boards to become more aware of their structure, functions, and their goals—that is, to *envision* what governance means. When we have accomplished these tasks, our boards will be better able to cope with the challenging environment we currently face and will lead us to the exhilarating promise of the era that awaits us.

"Boards must stay above the fray of daily organizational activities, look back at the total landscape and watch over the harbor of the organization's future."

FAYE WATTLETON
Former President,
Planned Parenthood Federation of America

CHAPTER ONE:

OVERVIEW

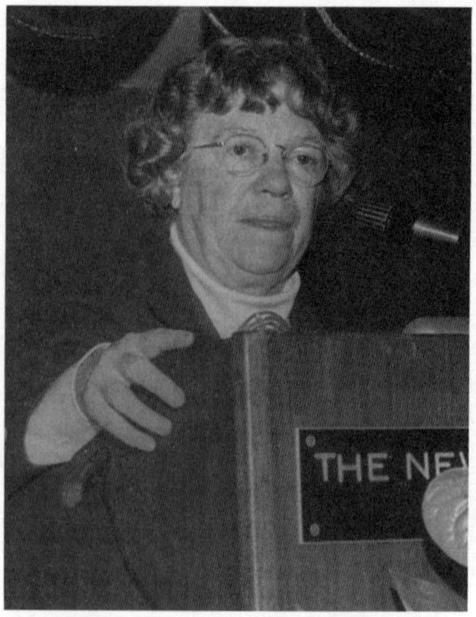

Margaret Mead speaking to the PPFA National Meeting in 1947.

"Never doubt that a small group of thoughtful, committed citizens can change the world. Indeed, it is the only thing that ever has."

MARGARET MEAD

Change. Above all else, this book is about change. In the 1980s, Planned Parenthood affiliates and the national office radically altered our financial base. We created public affairs entities to influence public policy and shape public opinion. We strengthened our ability to compete in the health care marketplace by improving productivity, developing marketing strategies, and diversifying service. And we tripled our capacity to attract private philanthropic dollars, using modern fund-raising techniques. Now we must devote the same energy and ingenuity to transforming our boards to contemporary, efficient work groups.

"In the Garden of Eden, Adam paused at one point and said: 'Eve, I believe we are going to be living in a time of great change.' The only stability that is predictable is the stability in constant change. Count on change. Plan on it."

JEROLD PANAS
Organization Consultant and Author

This book proposes a model and a rationale for change. It was conceived as a condensed reference that would synthesize organizational theory about boards for Planned Parenthood executive directors and boards of directors. I attempt to address ways of creating excellence in every aspect of board work. I also extend some ideas of several experts on boards, focusing on the organization of Planned Parenthood. Main topics include the following:

- problems that boards confront, including complex dilemmas (e.g., distinguishing between leadership and management; distinguishing between the roles of volunteer board members and paid staff; and distinguishing between governance and operations);
- responsibilities and roles of boards; and
- successful methods for leading and revitalizing boards and ways to take risks wisely.

In addition to providing general principles and suggestions, I include examples of board successes and difficulties, stories of actual experiences that have galvanized people in Planned Parenthood to go beyond the routine practices and the outworn models of the past.

Sources. Interspersed throughout the book are quotations from board experts and affiliate leaders, as well as extended examples of three affiliate boards in action. The quotations from affiliate leaders came directly from personal interviews that I conducted throughout 1989. Additionally, in 1988 I surveyed Planned Parenthood board presidents and executive directors throughout the country. Results from this survey, which had an excellent response rate of over 75 percent, are reported periodically in marginal side bars in this book when they relate to an issue being discussed. At the end of the book is a bibliography of books, pamphlets, newsletters, reports, and manuals that I consulted.* Additionally, these are all excellent references for those interested in the issues of voluntary leadership and the general subject of boards of directors.

Executive Summary. Since this book is meant to be a reference for affiliate leaders, the remainder of this chapter outlines the key concepts and the organization of this book. I hope that this will allow readers to locate topics and issues that are most pertinent to their own boards.

The FOREWORD explains briefly why Planned Parenthood

---

* Note: If a quotation appearing in my text or in marginal sidebars is not cited in the bibliography, it came from my interviews.

boards are so important and what they need to do to meet contemporary needs.

CHAPTER ONE, "Overview," introduces the phenomenon of organizational change. It also provides an overview of sources used in this book and summarizes the key points contained in each chapter.

CHAPTER TWO, "What Is the Problem with Boards?" describes typical problems confronted by boards. Organizational theorists and consultants confirm that boards have a difficult time with the following: focusing on the big picture and the bottom line; setting boundaries and ground rules to keep from meddling in staff business; and recruiting, and then retaining, talented board members. My own survey and interviews with selected affiliate leaders confirm that the difficulties that Planned Parenthood boards confront are the same ones that occur across the full spectrum of nonprofit organizations.

CHAPTER THREE, "The Duties and Roles of the Board," begins with the legal definition of board responsibility and the four statutory duties of all board members – the duties of care, loyalty, obedience, and diligence. It then describes the five roles the board plays in providing affiliate leadership. If Planned Parenthood boards do these five things well, they likely will succeed; if not, they will fail. The big five are: (1) plan *strategically* toward the future; (2) establish *policy* that guides the affiliate; (3) *supervise,* employ, and support a first-rate executive; (4) *advocate* for and champion the cause; and (5) *fund raise* to ensure that the affiliate has adequate private capital. In order to perform these roles well, most boards need to stop doing almost everything else.

Chapter Three concludes by suggesting that the language we have often used to describe boards fails us. Boards are not so much "directors" as they are "trustees" of our cause and "stewards" of our resources. Such matters are not merely haggling over semantics; the words we choose create our images and expectations.

CHAPTER FOUR, "The Board as Strategic Planner," describes the basic attributes of successful strategic plans. Namely, the plans that boards aim to develop and ratify should be broad; they produce profound impact if they are achieved; they pre-empt problems by anticipating; and they often propose initiatives that redirect the historical path of the affiliate. Boards too often get overwhelmed by the task of long-range strategic planning because they believe they must single-handedly create the plan. This is simply untrue; the executive director is the primary organizational planner. The board's planning job is best seen as reacting, responding to, and re-shaping staff proposals, and then owning the final product.

This chapter gives several caveats about long-range and strategic planning. The plan should focus on goals for some time in the future (e.g., five years) and should not simply extend into the future what exists in the present. Once plans have been made, boards should consult their plans repeatedly in making important decisions. Boards should generally avoid the temptation to interfere when the staff turns plans into reality. The chapter ends by describing some excellent planning documents already existing throughout the federation that may be helpful and time-saving. Following this chapter, "The Kalamazoo Story" is an extended description of how one affiliate, Planned Parenthood in Kalamazoo, survived a crisis, with particular attention to the ways in which planning influenced the process and the outcome.

CHAPTER FIVE, "The Board as Policy Setter," defines organizational policy and discusses the role of the board in setting policy. Ideally a board should establish policies on all matters of importance concerning the affiliate and then write and format these in a way that is easily retrievable. Staff can then use written policies to make the decisions necessary to implement them. Since policymaking can seem vague, this chapter contains examples of how one board, Planned Parenthood of Northern New England (PPNNE), has articulated policy in several critical areas, such as the board's relationship with the public; the authority that the board delegates to the executive director; and the board's organizational values and its financial policies (constraints and prohibitions). Following each policy example is a brief discussion of its practical implications.

CHAPTER SIX, "The Board as Boss," discusses the board's role as the employer of the executive director. The fact that this is not a classic supervisory relationship means that the board and the executive director should create clear and quantifiable results, e.g., affiliate service numbers, balance sheet financial ratios, and fund-raising goals that provide benchmarks to gauge executive performance. This chapter suggests ways of appraising the performance of the executive director and discusses briefly the issues of searching for and, if need be, terminating the executive director. This chapter ends with a strong plea that boards need to offer excellent salaries and benefit packages to gain or retain the caliber of managerial excellence necessary for an affiliate to succeed.

CHAPTER SEVEN, "The Board as Fund Raiser and Advocate," explores the last two board roles, arguing that the board must accept these functions of fund raising and advocacy for the affiliate to achieve success. One of the chief problems is that there have not been sufficient *structures* to organize the board properly. As an example of structures that may help, I describe two views that have been advanced within Planned Parenthood. The first is a model used by Doris Critz Yankee (a renowned Planned Parenthood fund-raising expert) that fully involves the board, giving each board member two committee assignments—a regular board committee *and* a fund-raising committee. The second model creates an advocacy structure developed by Anne Saunier (former chair of the PPFA board). This model proposes direct advocacy activism by each board member (rather than the board as recipient of staff briefings), and it also focuses attention on political issues and key elected officials. At the end of this chapter, "The Seattle Story" tells how the board of Planned Parenthood in Seattle rose to the occasion as both advocate and fund-raiser, illustrating how these two roles can complement each other.

CHAPTER EIGHT, "The Board Chair," turns from the discussion of the main board roles to focus on the critical issue of volunteer leadership, especially that of the board president. A sample job description for the board president emphasizes the three "R's": Requirements, Responsibilities, and Roles. The best style of leadership for Planned Parenthood presidents is identified as nonautocratic, with a knack of knowing how to blend process and task. An important leadership task of the president is to design and chair effective board meetings. This chapter discusses some desirable ways of doing this, including advance briefing and preparation for the president; a meeting plan that includes a diversity of subjects and of multiple presenters; use of efficiency techniques, especially time management; and the need to keep the board discussions from being monopolized by certain people (including the staff who attend). The chapter suggests how to orient new board presidents and how to avoid losing prematurely the sage advice of previous presidents.

CHAPTER NINE discusses "The Partnership: Board President and Executive Director." A good working relationship between the two bodes well for organizational health of the entire affiliate. The ideal is a shared power model that crisply identifies distinct areas of responsibility, with a shared leadership at its core. Both the president and the executive director should expect a hard-working partner and mutual respect. What the executive director needs most from the president is perspective, a willingness to fix board problems, a sense of equality, and a supportive employment setting. Likewise, presidents should be able to assume that their executive directors will strive for organizational excellence, provide accurate and timely information, and possess a true desire for a powerful board.

CHAPTER TEN, "Recommendation for Board Renewal and Board Structure," focuses on two major dynamics that can either bedevil a board or, if handled well, contribute to board success. The first subject is board renewal, which includes recruitment, retreat, and retention. Recruitment is the nomination and election of a steady, diverse, and talented cadre of new board members; retreat is the idea that boards must take time to get away from the myriad of short-term demands that compete for their attention and spend some uninterrupted quality time with each other. Retention is the capacity of boards to hold onto their members so that the organization can receive the "return on investment" and benefit from the wisdom that comes with experience.

The next subject relates to the need to structure the board in ways that accentuate the whole and control the parts. The time-honored approach of organizing the board into smaller work groups (committees) to work on specified functional areas (such as personnel) has for many nonprofits become part of the problem, not part of the solution. Permanent standing committees should be kept to a minimum and should reflect board responsibilities—not staff management areas. Whenever possible, boards should aim for temporary sub-structures that are fast-moving and that work as task forces and think tanks.

CHAPTER ELEVEN, "Making a Good Board Great: The Importance of Taking Risks Wisely," leads with the twin notions that boards, not circumstances, determine success, and that boards possess the power to make or break our affiliates. It is important for boards to fulfill their legal responsibilities and cope successfully with many dilemmas. However, boards should not get in a perpetual pattern of reacting defensively to problems. The question becomes this: How do boards make the transition from artful dodgers to pro-active policymakers—in other words, setting and accomplishing their own agendas? The secret to becoming an excellent board is to have the ability *to take risks for the right reasons,* while simultaneously building a series of safety nets just in case the decisions don't work out.

Taking risks and breaking new ground have always characterized our most distinguished affiliates. The chapter recommends ways for boards to simultaneously take risks and still be prudent. The approach is to: (1) diversify risk; (2) select endeavors that really matter; (3) prepare for risk by putting money in the bank; (4) find outside partners to share the risk; and (5) create an organizational culture that supports risk. The chapter ends with "The Vermont Story," which describes how the Planned Parenthood affiliate took an enormous risk in standing up to the Vermont state legislature, while simultaneously creating the programs, systems, and supports that made taking the risk a successful strategy.

In the AFTERWORD, guidance is given about key things to remember if a board wants to begin to reinvent itself, to better define and discharge its roles, to support its leadership, and to restructure its organization. The very best boards do *not* over-manage the affiliate's operations, but they *do* emphasize the following: making long-range plans, articulating values and policies, using time wisely, finding excellent board members and a first-rate executive director, and using the board deliberative process to fulfill their responsibilities and to seek innovative change.

CHAPTER TWO:

WHAT IS THE PROBLEM WITH BOARDS?

"Boards are:

- *awash in an endless stream of short-term matters and are not focused on the big goals, the basic values, the dreams;*
- *ineffective because the traditional things we ask boards to do are archaic, irrelevant and even if done well, often unnecessary; and*
- *lacking in the accountability to a bottom line that would focus their efforts."*

JOHN CARVER
Governance Consultant

A Truly Difficult Job. Voluntary boards are the backbone of a movement such as Planned Parenthood. As organizational leaders, we expect so much from voluntary boards that it is not surprising if we are sometimes disappointed. Even Boards of Planned Parenthood affiliates, which are often among the best of the nonprofit boards in communities, experience many difficulties. Boards are often inundated with so many tasks that it is difficult for them to succeed. Often boards are absorbed in reacting to short-term problems, maintaining the board itself, and keeping an eye on current operations. There is simply no time left in which to do the unique things that only a board can do.

Why does this happen? There are powerful tendencies that can easily direct boards:

- Reacting is easier than acting.
- Dealing with the here-and-now is easier than dealing with the future.
- Planning seems to be a luxury that boards cannot afford at times when their organizations are hanging on by their fingernails to survive.
- Overseeing operations is seen as the board's attempt to scrutinize staff to ensure that they are running programs in the same way as

the board would—as opposed to the task of determining whether the job is being done well or not.

If all of these dynamics are operating at the same time, boards can look very busy, pass many motions, pay the bills, and keep the organization's doors open. But they will fail to fulfill their role of visionary trustee.

When I interviewed a number of Planned Parenthood board leaders around the country, many of the people I spoke with gave the impression of being talented, competent, and devoted. Almost universally, they were enthusiastic about being involved in the work of Planned Parenthood, despite (or because of) the many external battles that the organization has faced in recent years at international, national, and local levels.

However, these board leaders were not always sure that their boards were getting the right things done in the best way possible. Sometimes their experiences were frustrating and not as rewarding as they had anticipated. Some talked of actual board uprisings and rebellions in which the board splintered into factions. Some spoke of executive directors who dominated the organization, while others complained about executive directors whose leadership skills were too weak.

In instances such as these—whatever the cause of the problem—it seems that once board members and staff became frustrated, the affiliate often tried to cope in a number of ways, such as:

- ignoring the possibility that board work could be done differently;
- waiting for super-president to come along and make it better;
- expecting too little because board members lead very busy lives and are, after all, just volunteers;
- politely and publicly touting one's great board but privately trashing the idea that a board is needed at all; and
- keeping the boards soothed with "feel good" staff presentations and catered lunches so members at least will feel guilty enough to raise a little money.

Such attitudes and actions often prove ultimately ineffective for the organization as a whole and frustrating for everyone involved. I found myself wondering why this was so: Why would a group of talented and motivated individuals assembled in a board of directors encounter such problems, and such difficulties in trying to resolve them?

Historical Roots. I first looked to my own professional experience. I have worked for Planned Parenthood for almost 18 years, over 15 as the executive director of an affiliate that now covers Maine, New Hampshire, and Vermont. I have also had the opportunity to consult with and provide workshops for over 40 Planned Parenthoods in every region of the United States and with affiliates of many types—large and small, urban and rural, weak and strong. Thus, I have been given the opportunity to observe and interact with boards and staff in action and in many diverse circumstances.

My impression is that some of the problems that affect Planned Parenthood boards today arise from changes that have occurred over time. The challenges that affiliate boards encountered in the 1970s were in some ways very different from the challenges of the 1990s. Some 20 years ago the managerial "professionalism" of the executive director (and often the senior staff) began to emerge. This became possible because of the major influx of government funds (primarily federal), providing resources that enabled Planned Parenthoods to offer extensive training to incumbents and to hire experienced managers (not just social workers, ministers, or nurses who did not always have such managerial preparation or experience). This trend continued for other senior staff positions. In my affiliate, for instance, our first finance director was a conscientious objector doing two years of community service; our next finance director had an MBA.

This development profoundly affected boards, because one of the board's basic jobs had been to provide the business or professional expertise that board members brought from "the real world." Even when staff began to have that expertise, many boards continued to behave and structure themselves as if they still had novices running the shop. This has often caused gridlock and role confusion.

Despite such changes, some of the same organizational issues from that earlier era look extremely familiar to many of us today. Who leads and who follows—the executive director or the board? How can a group of 25 people with a relatively "soft" hierarchy act efficiently and assertively to respond to an ever-changing world? Does a board dare to take risks when by legal duty, the board is conservator and steward of the resources? These remain compelling questions for Planned Parenthood affiliates and their boards.

My experience tells me that the solutions to Planned Parenthood board "problems" (i.e., opportunities in disguise) have for some time existed internally within the federation. One has only to look at any number of stellar boards that have helped to create affiliates of distinction and excellence. But before considering the wisdom of the achievers within our family, I wanted to enlarge the scope of my inquiry to see what the literature has to say about the current condition of nonprofit boards. This would help to answer the question of whether the difficulties encountered in some Planned Parenthood affiliates were unique to Planned Parenthood or were shared by other nonprofits.

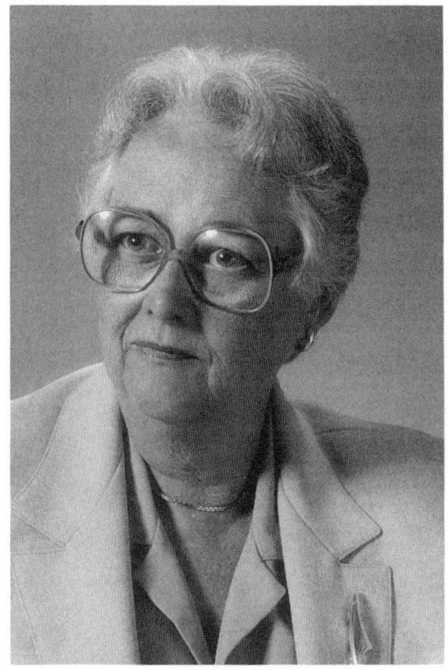

"Even great boards can be damaged by one destructive member. We once had a person who picked apart every committee recommendation—who wanted to re-enact every discussion at the Board meeting. That's hard on morale."

LEE MINTO
Executive Director
Planned Parenthood
of Seattle-King County

The Literature. In looking at books, journals, articles, and scholarly papers on the status of nonprofit boards, I found what seemed to be an emerging consensus that nonprofit boards were experiencing many of the same problems that were happening at Planned Parenthood.

Jennings, Hood and Associates, an organization specializing in work with nonprofit boards, states that the critical factors generally leading to poor performance by boards lie in six crucial activities:

- deficiencies in the selection process;
- lack of understanding of the board's duties and responsibilities;
- insufficient board education;
- failure to use the skills and talents that exist within the board;
- failure to communicate with and within the board; and
- the absence of an institutional long-range plan.

Another view comes to us from Howard Gesbeck, who has looked at the problems of nonprofit boards in behavioral terms. He found that boards:

- don't look at the big picture;
- don't operate in a business-like fashion and treat the organization as a business;
- don't split up the work well;
- don't purchase adequate liability insurance;
- too often allow one person to count all the eggs;
- attempt to do staff work;
- tolerate members missing board meetings; and
- too often sit silently.

Sheri Tepper, retired executive director of Rocky Mountain Planned Parenthood, defined some classic problem areas and labeled them as five "trouble signs" of boards gone astray:

- inaction and indecision;
- board meddling in program;
- cliquishness;
- sniping at staff; and
- lack of presidential management.

These are pervasive issues, but they are not peculiar to boards. They are often found when human beings attempt to work as a group. In order to solve these "group" problems, we must look for their underlying causes, which may include faulty structures, unrealistic expectations, and unclear roles. Without direction and reasonable expectations, people will inevitably respond badly, whether they are board members or staff members or members of an ice hockey team.

The Provocative John Carver. In the mid-1980s, some rather dramatic (to some, in fact, disturbing), ideas of board revitalization within the federation were being presented and discussed. Many of these were put forth by John Carver, a governance consultant who specializes in working with profit, nonprofit, and public organizations on the role and design of boards of directors. Carver provocatively painted a gloomy picture of boards of directors for the public sector and for nonprofit organizations who appeared to him to be frequently overworked, frustrated, and achieving little. To rectify this problem, he offered a new design or model of governance that helped boards focus on top priority concerns and made more efficient the overwhelming job of the board. H. Stanley Eichenauer was a member of a nonprofit board of directors that turned to Carver for help and improvement. In Eichenauer's view, after following the Carver principles, his board improved its accountability, productivity and quality of debate: "Changing how the board worked was difficult because . . . we grieved the loss of the familiar and prized ways of doing business. We are just as grateful that he (Carver) relentlessly pushed us to transform our governance process. As a result, our 'pseudo accountability' around trivia has been replaced by real accountability around major issues. Our retroactivity has yielded to pro-activity. Our slickness and uncontested yes-solutions have dissolved into enthusiastic and productive argument. Our organization is strongly poised to take on the future. Our constituency's values are well articulated and form the basis of our values."

> ***"We are so busy doing the urgent that we don't have time for the important."***
>
> **CONFUCIUS**

Carver shared his views with Planned Parenthood audiences at several national and regional meetings, facilitated some of the early meetings of the PPFA National Governance Task Force, and conducted training seminars with more than a dozen individual affiliates. Carver believes that nonprofit boards are failing, not because of a shortage of concerned and competent members, or a lack of staff support, but because boards "are awash in an endless stream of short-term matters and are not focused on the big goals, the basic values, the dreams."

Minor Repair or Major Overhaul? Carver sees board performance as punctuated with lost opportunity. Boards fail to achieve their potential, instead rubber-stamping and playing out ritual activities. But Carver does more than just lament this situation. His suggestions are as clear, crisp, and logical as a blueprint for a new facility.

The best way to understand Carver's ideas on boards is to read his

10 founding principles on governance, which appeared on the handout cover of his training notebook:

FIGURE ONE:

Carver's Commandments for Governing Boards

1. Govern pro-actively through explicit statements of values, rather than reactively or through event specific decisions; boards must be *at least* as disciplined as they expect their staffs to be.

2. Using four categories, address board values about:
- ENDS—what benefits for which needs are worth what cost
- STAFF MEANS—unacceptable practices and circumstances
- BOARD-STAFF LINK—how power is passed and accountability evaluated
- BOARD PROCESS—how the board will govern and on whose behalf

3. Spend most board time addressing ENDS with a long-term perspective; this is the board's major contribution to long-range planning.

4. Address STAFF MEANS only in a negative or constraining way in order to leave maximum freedom, but within clear limits.

5. Always resolve value issues starting with the largest, granting the CEO authority to decide all further (smaller) issues.

6. The board's job contributions or products *must* include:
- Linkage with the "ownership"
- Explicit governing values (policies)
- Assurance of executive performance

They may include other "values added," such as:
- Donor funding
- Legislative impact

7. The CEO position exists to accomplish ENDS without violating constraints on STAFF MEANS . . . and nothing else.

8. Routinize the monitoring of staff performance against all board policies on ENDS and STAFF MEANS, recognizing the measurement as *the* evaluation of CEO performance.

9. Official board committees, if any, are to help with the board's job, *never* with the staff's. Their best contribution is to prepare policy options (with implications) for board deliberation.

10. Use board time to create the future more than to review the past, to stimulate debate on ENDS rather than MEANS and to look outside the organization more than inside.

"I worry some about these new board models that streamline things and get very 'corporate.' Will we lose participation?"

ETHELYN BISHOP
Former PPFA Board Member and President of Planned Parenthood of Metropolitan Washington

Carver's proposals are not quick fixes or small, incremental changes, but are remarkable for what they say boards must do, and what they must stop doing. He proposes very small boards (e.g., over seven members should only happen with some compelling justification) without any direct involvement in either budgets or personnel policies. Is this heretical? Irresponsible? Unrealistic? Some who worked with these rather radical notions are convinced that they *can* work, and that furthermore, one need not use all the ideas but could choose and adapt those that most appeal to an individual board's current condition, historic culture, and sense of priorities.

Carver's ideas have become a catalyst for much discussion on the subjects of boards, their relationship with the executive director, and the notion that there must be a better way. Not everyone, however, agrees with Carver's ideas. Norah Holmgren, PPFA Western Region, remembers it this way: "Carver's critics found his work idiosyncratic and his language riddled with jargon. His theories seemed to be still evolving and incomplete. His total preoccupation with bottom-line results seemed to ignore the fact that nonprofits had a more holistic model of success and couldn't so neatly separate means and ends. His ideas on monitoring and evaluation didn't seem to be workable." Whether one enthusiastically endorsed or criticized what he had to say, Carver had touched a vital nerve within the Planned Parenthood family. His ideas focused attention on key issues and challenged the conventional wisdoms of what boards must do or should never do. Certain affiliates, as well as the national board itself, have begun experimenting with major changes of board structure, content, form, and function.

> ***"As a passionate leader, I like Carver's ideas on governance precisely because they are so passionless. His model gives the board rules that, when used fairly, makes us efficient enough to have the time to again be passionate."***
>
> **ANNE SAUNIER**

Too Little Time, Too Much to Do. The biggest problem that most boards face is finding enough time in order to be successful. The second biggest problem is figuring out the right number of people required to get the job done. It would be wrong to suggest that the numbers reported on page 24 (figure two) should be construed as the ideals for which affiliates should shoot. But an affiliate might find it useful to compare its own performance results against these federation-wide averages and see if any major discrepancies exist. If a board is having a problem in an area that might be impacted by size, number of committees, or frequency of meetings, this table may give that board some guidelines for improvement.

This baseline information regarding how much working time the board has raises some interesting questions. For instance, the average board of a Planned Parenthood affiliate meets *just under 20 hours a year*—or about half of one regular business work-week. Does this provide enough

FIGURE TWO:

In 1988 the Average Size of Planned Parenthood Boards and Average Frequency of Meetings

Number of board members	27
Number of board committees	8
Length of board meetings	2.16 hours
Number of board meetings per year	9
Length of committee meetings	1.56 hours
Number of committee meetings per year	40

time for the board to govern the agency? There is no simple answer to this question. But at the very minimum, it suggests that boards do not spend very much time at the crucial group decision point – the board meeting itself. This will become a problem unless every minute at the board meeting is used wisely.

Summing Up. The board experts whose ideas I've reported used very different ways to analyze the performance of boards. But the fundamental thread that ran through their critiques was that boards have a very hard time with their central role – namely, *making policy decisions that advance the organization toward achieving its mission.* Jennings, Hood and Associates called this deficit ". . . the absence of an institutional long-range plan." Gesbeck's observation was that boards failed to " . . . look at the big picture" and "on the big goals, the basic values, the dreams." Tepper described the board's problem as "one of . . . inaction and indecision."

What does this view – that boards have difficulty achieving their mission, given constraints on available time and people – mean for the boards of Planned Parenthood? I believe that while most Planned Parenthood boards can't work much harder, they can work much smarter to enable them to reach their goals more easily. The way to do this is to focus 80 percent of board time on: (1) planning strategically, (2) setting corporate policy, (3) supervising the chief executive officer, (4) advocating for the cause, and (5) fund raising private dollars. If boards will rivet their attention on these five tasks, there will be enough time to govern the organization, and they will be making their unique contribution to affiliate success.

CHAPTER THREE:

THE DUTIES AND ROLES OF THE BOARD

The Basics. Why do Planned Parenthood affiliates have boards at all? The *Board Officer's Manual,* written by Patty Boyle and Norah Holmgren from the PPFA Western Region Office, says it with elegant simplicity. "Every nonprofit organization must have a board of directors. It's a legal requirement. A nonprofit corporation is presumed to be acting in the public's interest and must therefore have public representation in its decision-making. Board volunteers give the organization the authority to act. They legitimize the organization." As with many other things in life, if the Internal Revenue Service requires it, one does it.

> *"In the eyes of the law, there is no such thing as a dummy or nominal board of directors. The law confines the business of management of a corporation to its directors and they are vested with fiduciary duty to participate actively and fully in the management of corporate affairs."*
>
> **THE MINNESOTA SUPREME COURT**

> *" First things first . . . And other things not at all."*
>
> PETER DRUCKER

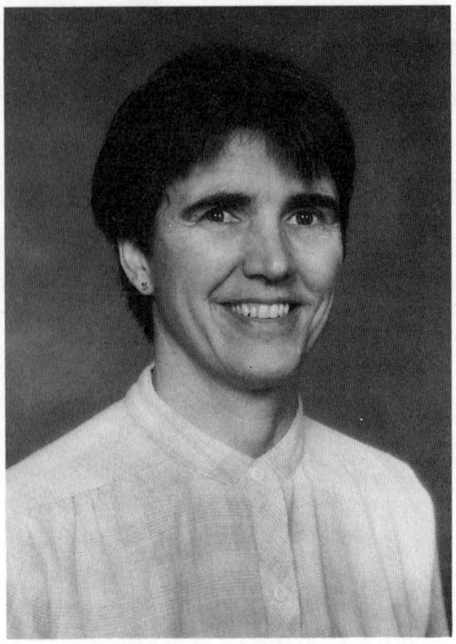

"Board members fulfill the nonprofit role of meeting with the public trust. If the community believes in the board, then they'll believe that their money is being spent right."

CATHY FRANK
PPFA Board Member and Former President of Planned Parenthood of Northern New England

In truth, the legal requirement perfectly captures the ethical and logical response to why boards should exist. Boards are not self-interested (i.e, paid for their work), but are instead interested in the public good and community benefits of Planned Parenthood's programs. They seek to provide the perspective of the stake-holders they represent: clients, donors, and public officials. By participating on the board, an individual lends the credibility of his/her name and reputation.

Duties: Legal Responsibilities of Individual Board Members. In the fall of 1991, PPFA published a two-page brochure titled *Board Responsibility* that captures the generic duties (from a legal, corporate statutory basis) of board members. This brochure describes the three duties as:

- DUTY OF CARE – Board members are expected to act in good faith. They must use the same care that a reasonably prudent person in a similar position would use in like circumstances.

- DUTY OF LOYALTY – Board members must act in the best interests of the organization and must not engage in activities that would hurt the corporation or engage in self-dealing. There must be no conflict of interest between their professional obligations to the organization and their personal interests. If a potential conflict exists, it is necessary that the conflict be identified and disclosed, and an appropriate manner of response be adopted.

- DUTY OF OBEDIENCE – Directors and officers are expected to act in accordance with applicable state and federal laws, as well as in accordance with the organization's articles of incorporation and bylaws. There is a myriad of regulations that may pertain to the organization. It is incumbent on the board to ensure that the organization remains abreast of all applicable laws.

Additionally, the text goes on to describe what I would identify as a fourth legal duty:

- DUTY OF DILIGENCE – Any actions taken by a board must reflect the fact that the board has carefully reviewed all relevant information and made an informed decision. Lawyers, accountants, and others with specific expertise should be consulted when appropriate. To ensure thoughtful decision making, it is important that board members attend meetings and be well pre-

> pared to address all issues of relevance to the organization. Accurate minutes detailing board deliberations, actions taken and resolutions passed must be kept. Minutes should be closely reviewed by all board members and corrections noted. If a board member has been absent and disagrees with an action taken, the board member should, in writing, outline his/her position.

Thus, we have the bedrock responsibilities and duties of all board members spelled out in legal terms. As the board solves its problems, discharges its roles, and provides leadership, it must always bear in mind the four legal and fiduciary obligations listed here. Simply put, to do less could be illegal.

But after the board has assured itself that these minimum requirements are being accomplished, it is left with the central dilemma of this book. Namely, how does the board provide value-added vision, imagination, and creativity in the 20 or so hours allotted annually for deliberation and debate? The process starts with unswerving allegiance to the essence of Drucker's admonition that leads off this chapter, ". . . first things first, and others not at all." In other words, boards must stick to a handful of roles – done in depth, done with proven techniques, and done with regularity. All else must wait.

Boards have little margin for error in how they use their time. Staying in role and staying on task are the essential elements for success. The five-point, star-shaped model pictured on page 28 seems to me the best way to define the roles of a Planned Parenthood board: strategic planner, policy setter, supervisor of the CEO, fund raiser, and advocate. Clearly, there is nothing revolutionary about this five-point description. None of these roles would likely be disputed by experts on the subject of board governance, although some organizational experts would most likely produce a longer, more complicated and fancier-sounding list of board duties. The utility of the five-point description is its reductive simplicity. It points out five areas within the organization for which the board takes primary responsibility.

Some board members may panic when they first hear about this virtually exclusive focus on five main roles. What about all the other things that boards do? What about passing budgets, ratifying personnel policies, and monitoring programs? Not to worry. John Carver points out that if board decisions in its main areas truly set organizational direction, a chain reaction occurs. Board macro-decisions allow (in fact, require) staff to make hundreds of smaller operational decisions. If the board's strategies and policies are dynamic and visionary, they will propel the organization down a path of strength, growth, and

FIGURE THREE:

All Nonprofit Boards Begin as a Pyramid

A Planned Parenthood Board Must Become a Star

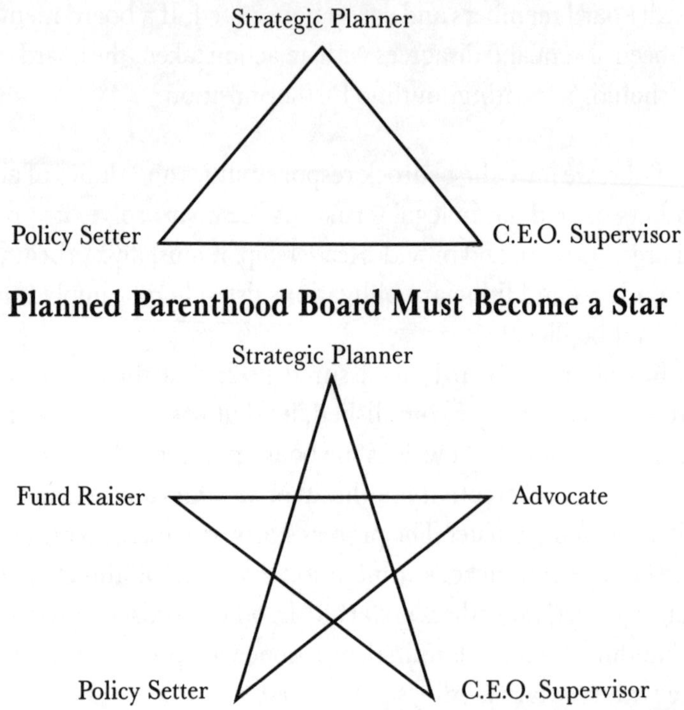

success. Conversely, if the board's decisions in these areas are shallow, inconclusive, and immersed in detail, they still will propel the organization into activity—but it will be like a Rube Goldberg contraption that spins and whirs but goes nowhere.

Strategic planning, policy development, supervision of the C.E.O., advocacy for our cause, and fund raising are universal needs for all Planned Parenthoods. The job of the board is not merely to check off whether these tasks have been completed, but also to make sure that they are being done well, generating outstanding products and mapping out successful outcomes. Long-term performance results define a board's effectiveness. Fortunately, easily adapted techniques and methods already are practiced by the best affiliate boards, so that other boards do not need to re-invent the wheel and waste valuable time and energy.

Getting to the Heart of the Matter. What exactly should the Planned Parenthood board do and what should it avoid doing in order to do its job well? We must continue to remember that the board exists as an assembled decision-making body for an average of only 20 hours per year, which is equivalent to half a work-week. What the board does and what it must avoid doing are both important. Priority-setting is everything, as organizational expert, Peter Drucker, advises, "first things first . . . and others not at all."

When boards break down and become dysfunctional, it is usually because they are trying to do too much; they try to oversee the entire operation. And by accepting this unrealistic expectation, boards end up accomplishing far too little. John Carver reminds us that boards should not and cannot do "everything that *is important* to an agency." There is not enough time, even if the board wanted to involve itself in every critical organizational activity. Staying disciplined and focused is the trademark of an effective board.

The Five Things a Board Must Do. Please excuse the apparent redundancy, but the truth bears repeating. Planned Parenthood boards have five basic duties or roles. Although some of these duties are shared with the executive director, the buck stops with the board. If boards do only these five things, do them well, and eliminate everything else, most Planned Parenthood affiliates will improve dramatically their effectiveness. Again, the five board duties are:

- PLAN STRATEGICALLY toward the future;
- ESTABLISH POLICY that guides the affiliate and articulates the values that frame these future strategies;
- SUPERVISE, employ, and support a first-rate executive;
- ADVOCATE for and champion the Planned Parenthood cause; and
- FUND RAISE to ensure that the affiliate has enough discretionary private capital to be financed properly in the present and future.

It may be comforting to see that there are only five major tasks for any board, but these are five of the most difficult and elusive endeavors that face our boards.

Think of your own board's last few meetings. How much time was spent in making decisions in these critical areas? Although these tasks are well known, they seem to be accomplished by only a handful of our best boards. Often, these duties become mere abstractions, and even if they are being implemented, success is difficult to measure. Another possible frustration is that being successful in four of the five tasks still can add up to zero. For example, an affiliate that lacks a long-range plan can be undone even if its board is doing an admirable job on the other four tasks.

Despite these difficulties, the boards that are squarely leading their affiliates by dealing with the important, strategic issues of our mission, by necessity concentrate on the big five because the stakes are too high if they do not. Bluntly put, exemplary risk-taking boards must stay ahead of the competition and opposition and must plan strategically because they have opted for future scenarios where both threat and opportunity loom. They must craft policy because the world moves fast and staffs need guidance. They must possess a first-rate executive director because the business operation is complex and requires the attention of an accomplished professional. They must advocate for Planned Parenthood's cause because they have inserted themselves as visible leaders in a body politic that will attempt to crush them. They will fund raise because in the current climate, private dollars are not merely the icing on the cake, but are essential to underwriting most new ventures.

Conversely, boards that have been ducking the strategic leadership of our times will slip into the conservative, safe harbor of reacting, monitoring, and maintaining. They may argue that the best they can do is survive, and that some day, somehow, when they get past the current crises, they'll start doing what they are supposed to do. But it will never happen, because if the job is defined as a maintenance position, it's a never-ending cycle. First, one thing breaks, and then another, and it becomes increasingly difficult to break old habits and get ahead of the game.

A Sixth Point to the Star? Many of our very best affiliates use their boards for a sixth primary function: the provision of unpaid technical expertise. Each board member is recruited for a particular area of knowledge. For example, the board may be composed of an investment banker, an architect, a computer expert, a planned giving specialist, a city planner, and a gynecologist. The expectation is that these persons will contribute their professional expertise as board "consultants" in certain relevant projects consistent with their background. The affiliate benefits because board members possess skills that would be very expensive in the marketplace. When this works, the results can be quite spectacular.

"Why boards are so important is pretty simple—a collection of heads is better than one."

LEE MINTO

However, sometimes this "bonus" can backfire, because it blurs distinctions that can be important. If, for example, the architect on the board chairs the Facility Committee for planning a new building, and the executive director discovers that the design ideas are not working, a thorny dilemma arises. If this were just the project architectural "consultant," the executive director could fire him or her. But the executive director can't fire the boss. There probably isn't an executive director who hasn't occasionally sought legal advice from a lawyer on the board or audit recommendations from a C.P.A. on the board. But to actually engage board members as informal consultants in operational activities is probably best left to affiliates that are already very strong and that have boards that are successful first and foremost on the big five. Unfortunately, it is often the weaker affiliates that use this approach because they simply can't afford to turn down volunteer help. Generally, however, expertise either should be possessed by the staff or obtained outside the organization. Boards are not adjuncts to staff; their role is specialized and unique. Obscuring that distinction invites failure.

Reconceptualizing Boards by Examining the Language We Use to Describe Boards. The words used in talking about boards are telling and powerful. They shape and perpetuate our expectations about what boards are supposed to do. Some of these words and the impressions they convey about boards may be outdated and in need of change if they are to reflect the reality of contemporary governance.

According to *The American Heritage Dictionary,* a board is an "organized body of administrators," and directors are individuals who "supervise, control, or manage." If we combine these definitions, a "board of directors" is a group of administrators or managers who supervise. This definition sounds suspiciously like a description of the role of staff and, if taken literally, it can be confusing, inaccurate, and much too ambitious and overreaching. Some Planned Parenthood affiliates have a great many programmatic and administrative affairs and multimillion dollar budgets. They also have boards that meet for an average of only 20 hours per year. That is not enough time to manage; it is barely enough time to govern. The world of nonprofit organizations has changed, and our affiliates should not be viewed as old-fashioned charities with a paid general secretary and a group of community fathers who manage the activities of social service staff.

> ***"Good stewardship means protecting and managing the donor's investment—so that it produces the best possible return. It means using the money as the donor intended it to be used."***
>
> **JAMES GREGORY LORD**

Perhaps the words that better convey the contemporary sense of what a nonprofit board does are "steward," "trustee," and "fiduciary." As a *steward,* the board manages the property and other assets of an absent ownership, a body composed of consumers, donors, or taxpayers. As *trustee,* the board is chosen to administer the affiliate's policy and funds on behalf of a beneficiary (the public good). As a *fiduciary,* the board exists not to benefit its individual members, but to protect and hold in trust the values and solvency of the stakeholder's interest in the organization, including clients, donors, and government officials. Overall, then, an affiliate board is a body of trustees who govern, inspire trust, and act as steward for the affiliate's assets, with a fiduciary responsibility for achieving the mission of Planned Parenthood.

Conclusion. Board members may end up gasping for breath after going through the litany of things required to achieve excellence as a strategic planner, policy maker, C.E.O. supervisor, fund raiser, and advocate. If that isn't enough, individual board members also must perform its legal duties. And then there are the expectations of steward, trustee, and fiduciary. How could any board do all this and at this level of involvement? It is important to note that these expectations are somewhat idealized and that boards will not be 100 percent successful in all areas, all of the time. Also, it takes time to reach top performance in each function, and it is impossible for a board to excel in these five functions as described and hold onto all the other things that it may have done in the past.

But imagine what an affiliate could accomplish if its board just did these five things. (Nothing else. No exceptions.) By giving up all the other distractions, would its effectiveness in the big five be doubled? My conjecture is that not only would the affiliate suffer no harm, but its performance would soar. The executive director would be held to a high standard of accountability. Staff would become more productive. And the affiliate would become a power within the federation.

Let's now move forward and look at how each of these five roles can be accomplished with vigor, vision, and ingenuity.

CHAPTER FOUR:

THE BOARD AS STRATEGIC PLANNER

"In planning, the board is more adviser than expert. The key for the executive director is to have educated the board well enough so they can give good advice."

CATHY FRANK

Planning is a crucial board responsibility, yet boards are often tempted to avoid it, either by going through the motions of planning dutifully but ineffectively, or by chronically postponing it. This happens in part because the assignment to plan can be a vague one, with no exact guidelines as to how to accomplish it and no scoring system to tell you if you have done it poorly or well. Without a clear sense of purpose, long-range and strategic planning can become merely a jargon-ridden exercise of interminable process and limited results. Planning also gets short shrift because it is difficult and takes time. In his *Strategic Planning Handbook,* Vaughn Keller has captured this point: "planning . . . encroaches upon managers as a distraction from the urgent demands of the present . . . an exercise in fantasy reserved for those who have the temperament and free time to engage in speculation." With this common attitude, planning seems to be a luxury rather than a necessity.

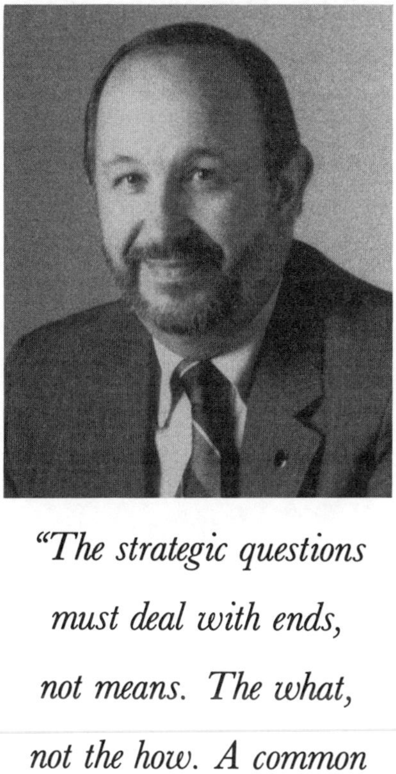

"The strategic questions must deal with ends, not means. The what, not the how. A common dilemma for boards in planning is to become mired in the details of implementation."

MARK SALO
Executive Director
Planned Parenthood of San Diego and Riverside Counties

> *"The primary benefit of the planning process is the process itself, and not a plan."*
>
> **GEORGE A. STEINER**

The Board as Strategic Planner. It is important for boards to remember why planning is vital. Common sense dictates that the best way to head into the future is to know where you want to go and to create a road map of how to get there. Furthermore, good planning helps one anticipate future events so one can outdo the competition and outwit the opposition.

It is not the role of board members to *initiate* the bold strokes of grand plans; often they simply do not have the time, or sometimes the expertise. The executive director MUST be the principal organizational planner. The board's role is better understood with the following in mind:

- consider which proposed staff alternatives advance the mission furthest;
- establish criteria by which to rank alternatives;
- determine whether proposals match the affiliate core values;
- help free staff from getting swamped with details.

The board's planning job often is simply to nudge staff back onto the pathway of appropriate dreams. While boards are reactors, they must not be passive. The board's job is to decide to pursue some things and discard others, and to ask the tough questions.

After a proposed set of solutions or actions has been debated and adopted, the board plays its important role of *owning the plan.* Although the board most likely has not been the primary architect or builder of the plan, the board is absolutely the primary owner of the plan. And, like a physical structure, the plan must be maintained with pride and renovated as needed. Owning a plan means returning to it when the organization hits a crisis. It means investing the "sweat equity" of capital fund raising if the plan calls for a new building; it means having the evaluation of the executive director based in part on accomplishment of the long-range objectives laid out in the plan.

Board Planning versus Staff Planning. There is an old leadership development caveat (I first heard it in a speech by management expert Warren Bennis) that goes something like this: "Management's job is to make sure that the organization does the *things right.* The board's job is to make sure the organization does the *right things.*" And selecting the right things for the organization's future is the heart of board planning. As Mark Salo asserts in the quotation at the beginning of the chapter, board planning is synonymous with strategic planning. It focuses on the ends and not the means. It searches for the what and leaves it to staff to figure out the how.

"Traditional long-range *planning is an administrative tool. Predictions are made on the basis of past performance, current resources and demographic trends.*

Strategic *planning is an entrepreneurial process. The organization attempts to* design *its own future—based on the external environment, its opportunities and constraints."*

JAMES GREGORY LORD

Strategic planning focuses on the forest, not the trees. It involves assessing the internal strengths and weaknesses of the affiliate. It looks at the big themes and powerful trends (e.g., economic, demographic, political, technological) at play in society. Taking into account these matters, boards attempt to forecast the opportunities and threats that the external environment will present. Good strategic planning decisions shore up weaknesses and optimize strengths on the inside of the organization, while vanquishing threats and seizing opportunities in the outside world.

And what are the issues that seem to be of strategic importance in the business of Planned Parenthood as we enter the decade of the 90s? I can't imagine a quality board plan that doesn't address national health care insurance, the AIDS epidemic, the shift of the abortion rights struggle to all 50 states, the possibility that the birth control pill might become an over-the-counter drug, or the trend away from single category health providers to managed care systems. Good board strategies go beyond just describing these societal dynamics; they choose future courses of action that position the affiliate to achieve its mission despite these issues or even because of these issues.

"Planning is a process that writes the script for the organization for a specific period of time."

VAUGHN KELLER

Six Planning Caveats. It is difficult to know where to begin on long-range, strategic planning. Boards invariably have questions about how to scan the environment for meaningful trends, how far into the future to go, and whether to redebate the articulation of the central purpose (e.g., mission) of the organization. There may be confusion as to how tightly the affiliate's plan must conform to the federation's and how explicitly the board must go in providing enough direction to enable staff to implement the plan. The following six procedures and principles can prove useful.

> ***"Simply reacting to the present demand or scrambling because of tensions is the opposite [of thoughtful planning]. Planning emphasizes conscious, disciplined choice."***
>
> **VAUGHN KELLER**

1. GET BEYOND THE PRESENT—DON'T AUTOMATICALLY LET TODAY'S REALITY DICTATE TOMORROW'S PLAN. Sometimes the first steps in planning are too closely meshed with current realities (e.g., "We don't have enough money to do this," or "Our community is too conservative for that"). These constraints may not apply in the future, but they may cause the board to get bogged down with detail and expend too much energy coping with the status quo. When this happens, the plan invariably settles for less than what is best. To counter this tendency, try this approach. Pick a time—three, five, or ten years into the future—and have the board describe where they want the affiliate to be. Then, work backward from the end point to the present. Thus, if the board has chosen a five-year time frame, the first goals listed are for year five, not next year. This technique, called "back planning," allows the organization to pick an outcome (e.g., "in five years, contraceptive services will have increased by 92 percent"), that often is bolder than it otherwise might be. Working backward from year five to the present frees up creativity.

2. BOARD PLANNING LOOKS FOR QUANTUM LEAPS, NOT INCREMENTAL CREEPS. Do not plan by simply extending what you are doing today to some fixed point in the somewhat distant future. If an affiliate is in a little trouble now, automatically doing five percent more per year may get it into even more trouble. For example, simply serving five percent more birth control patients per year who can't pay for their care may only put your budget further in the hole. Many of the strategic initiatives in a board plan should be geometric, not incremental. Figure four on page 37 illustrates this point.

3. USE THE BOARD FOR MISSION CONTROL. As established earlier in this chapter, board work should focus on planning a broad vision—THE WHAT. There is one additional area that is the province of the board—namely, the crucial question of WHY the organization exists. This primary "why" question should be given in a mission statement, which should eloquently capture the central purpose or reason-for-being of the organization. The mission statement also should be simple, understandable, and short (e.g., 100 words is bad, 25 better, and five best). For a very long time, many Planned Parenthoods lived with the mission statement, "Every child a wanted child." Most affiliates have moved beyond this because it didn't seem to capture the totality of why we exist and for whom we exist. Yet its clarity and power are seldom matched.

FIGURE FOUR:

Two Methods of Increasing Fund-Raising Revenue

Facts: A hypothetical affiliate has 1,000 donors and the average gift size is $50

Goal: To create a five year goal to increase fund raising

APPROACH ONE (INCREMENTAL): Through additional direct solicitation affiliate wants to increase gift size by five percent each year for five years. The following forecast is made.

Year One	– 1000 donors x 52.50 gift =	$ 52,500
Year Two	– 1000 donors x 55.12 gift =	55,120
Year Three	– 1000 donors x 57.87 gift =	57,870
Year Four	– 1000 donors x 60.76 gift =	60,760
Year Five	– 1000 donors x 63.80 gift =	63,800
Net total five year fund-raising revenue		$290,050

APPROACH TWO (STRATEGIC): Through additional direct solicitation affiliate wants to increase gift size by five percent each year for five years and additionally wants to triple the number of donors immediately. The following forecast is made.

Year One	– 3000 donors x 52.50 gift =	$157,500
Year Two	– 3000 donors x 55.12 gift =	166,500
Year Three	– 3000 donors x 57.87 gift =	173,610
Year Four	– 3000 donors x 60.76 gift =	182,280
Year Five	– 3000 donors x 63.80 gift =	191,400
Total five year fund-raising revenue		$871,290
Minus acquisition costs		-100,000
Net total five year fund-raising revenue		$771,290

Approach One forecasts increasing the fund-raising goal by making the average gift to the affiliate five percent higher for five straight years, while holding onto a donor base of 1000 contributors. Thus, the affiliate would be raising 28 percent more annually at the end of five years (a little higher than 25 percent through the magic of compound interest). But let's look at Approach Two. In this strategy, the affiliate invests $100,000 in year one with an aggressive direct-mail donor acquisition campaign, with the goal being to triple the number of donors. Let's say the affiliate is successful in acquiring the 2,000 new donors and also manages to raise all donors the annual five percent increase—the same outcome sought in the first approach. In the second scenario, the affiliate raises over 283 percent more money in year five by having made the up-front investment. Additionally, over the five years, the second approach raises 481,240 more dollars—even after subtracting the $100,000 donor acquisition cost. This is geometric, quantum-leap growth. It simply required laying out $100,000 up-front, which in this hypothetical plan provided results that were almost three times better because the money was invested at the beginning. It meant using a planning strategy (e.g., crafty thinking) that would significantly change the future by doing something different in the present.

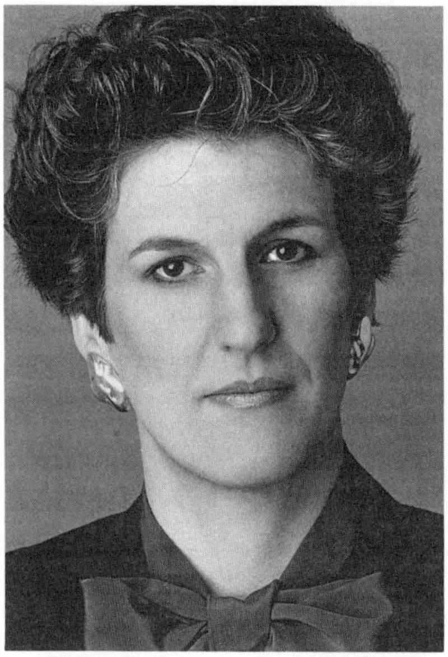

"This may sound heretical, but I don't see boards getting involved in long-range planning—at least the way planning is often practiced. I see the board focusing on values, those things we would never sacrifice and trying to see out, let's say, 10 years and establish the ends we want to achieve.

ANNE SAUNIER

Board debates on reviewing mission can be exciting and creative, or dull and lifeless. The revisiting of mission should be the first step in the strategic planning process. Here are suggestions to keep the process lively and pertinent:

"The mission statement has to be understandable. If a grade schooler can read, comprehend, and explain the statement, you are probably on the right track. You have performed well as a trustee!"

JEROLD PANAS

- Gather many examples of corporate mission statements—your current one, several of the most different from other affiliates, and several from the private sector. Comparing and contrasting will stretch the possibility of change.

- Create a list of the possibilities for new programs that the affiliate will consider in the planning process. It usually turns out to run the gamut from mobile vans to child care to adoption services. Now, look at the current mission statement and determine if these ideas will fit under your current central purpose (mission). If not, is the mission too narrow or is the program idea simply outside it?

- Look at last year's state legislative agenda and analyze some of the proposed statutes that the affiliate supported or was asked to support. Consider how that action fits with your current mission statement. For example, would your current mission enable you to take a stand on gay rights, equal pay proposals, or family leave statutes?

- Resist trying to rewrite the mission statement at the full board meeting. You'll get "group speak" and frustration. Use the collective thinking of the board to brainstorm organizational purpose, but don't turn it into a group-writing project.

4. BOARD PLANNING MUST AVOID GRIDLOCK. As this chapter establishes, board planning is fundamentally concerned with the mission statement, core values, and strategic outcome goals. But all too often, an affiliate's long-range plan resembles the "work plans" used in many corporate settings. The format is usually a grid sheet. On the horizontal axis are listed activities to be accomplished, the person or department responsible, target dates, ways to measure progress, and the cost budgeted to perform the task. On the vertical axis, each of the affiliate's goals and objectives is listed. Clearly, having tactics and objectives to undergird vision and strategy is necessary. But the board's job is to make sure the C.E.O. does it, not to try to do it themselves.

5. EXPECT THE PLAN TO BE DOG-EARED. Do not let plans

gather dust in a corner. Boards should revisit the major features of their strategic plan on a regular schedule, at least every other year. Do a planning exercise at almost every board meeting so that contemplating the future remains a lively, contemporary, and flexible task. Use your strategic plan as a benchmark when proposing your annual budget—e.g., evaluate the progress the affiliate has achieved on its long-range goals and appraise next year's budget against where your plan indicated you wanted to be.

6. BORROW IDEAS FROM THE VERY BEST PLANS. Start with and use other planning documents that have been produced by other affiliates and the federation. The current PPFA Strategic Plan can be a cornerstone; regional offices can supply prototype plans from other affiliates; the Metropolitan Executive Director's Council's *Planned Parenthood 2000* is filled with planning principles and ideas. Being part of a larger family of independent affiliates lets us build on some of the planning work done by our Planned Parenthood colleagues. Beyond generic planning models and texts, great planning aids specifically tailored to Planned Parenthood are available. Here are several I've found:

   - *Planning For the Future: A Guide for Planned Parenthood Boards* by Lee Minto (Seattle: Planned Parenthood of Seattle-King County, 1983). This six-page workbook is clear and brief. It defines the principal planning terminology and provides a step-by-step process. For some, the model advanced here gets into staff operational planning steps, and affiliates must decide for themselves how deeply to involve the board in each and every step.

   - *A Not-For-Profit Planning Model* by Mark Salo (San Diego: Planned Parenthood of San Diego and Riverside Counties, 1991). This 10-page document provides a method of planning. It also talks about the importance of framing the issues correctly, the key need for leaders to keep leading during the planning process, and the way in which group process can distort purposeful planning if allowed to go unchecked. Salo exposes a fatal flaw in many board long-range planning approaches. Namely, the board is brought together and an outside planning consultant facilitates and extracts a planning consensus from the group. Salo argues persuasively that the facilitation needs to come primarily from the formal leadership (board president, executive director, board officers) and informal leaders (the most knowledgeable and capable board

> ***"Strategic planning is innovative, exploratory, venturesome, and visionary. Impatient with convention, the success-driven organization is attracted by the unknown and the undetermined. There must be a declaration of an overriding goal to greatness."***
>
> **JEROLD PANAS**

members). The model is not specifically long-range—in fact, the time frame is yearly—but it is indeed visionary and strategic.

- *Strategic Planning Handbook* by Vaughn Keller (New York: Planned Parenthood Federation of America, 1983). This comprehensive workbook is targeted for Planned Parenthood affiliates. Keller is an organizational consultant who previously worked for PPFA as a management trainer and continues to work with several affiliates, especially in strategic planning. While this book's length and scholarly terminology can be challenging, it is a *must* for all executive directors, board presidents, and chairs of planning committees. It is loaded with planning techniques, caveats, and applications from the corporate world.

- *Resource Development System: A Process for Non-profit Organizations to Develop Effective Plans, Orchestrate Resources and Motivate Constituencies,* created by the Peat, Marwick Group. Some PPFA leaders were exposed to the Resource Development System in workshops sponsored by the PPFA Leadership Institute. This is an elaborate, focused approach that is probably best suited for the experienced affiliate that has already established a successful planning track record. Its strength is the combination of planning, resource development, and marketing on a strategic level.

Each of these references is available for order from the PPFA regional offices in San Francisco, Chicago, and Atlanta.

Planning with a Pyramid. A helpful way to conceptualize an affiliate's plan is to think of it as a four-layered pyramid as pictured in figure five. The image of a pyramid works on several levels. Overall, it suggests that a plan that will work must possess a broad, secure foundation grounded on the bedrock of reality (objectives). The component at the top will have the fewest words (and be most general), while each successive layer will require more words (and be more specific). There is a structural integrity and interdependence among the four layers: the *mission* defines the central purpose of the organization and answers the question of why the affiliate exists; the *principles* outline the core beliefs of the organization; the *goals/strategies* answer the question of what are we planning to do; and the *objectives/tactics* describe planned operational activities and how the goals are going to be achieved.

As suggested earlier, the board and the executive staff work together at the top three layers. The management staff takes on increasing

"The board of directors must also evaluate responsiveness to new situations. Planning is important, but organizations must reserve some time and resources for responding to new opportunities and unanticipated needs."

G. NEIL KARN

FIGURE FIVE:

Planning with a Pyramid

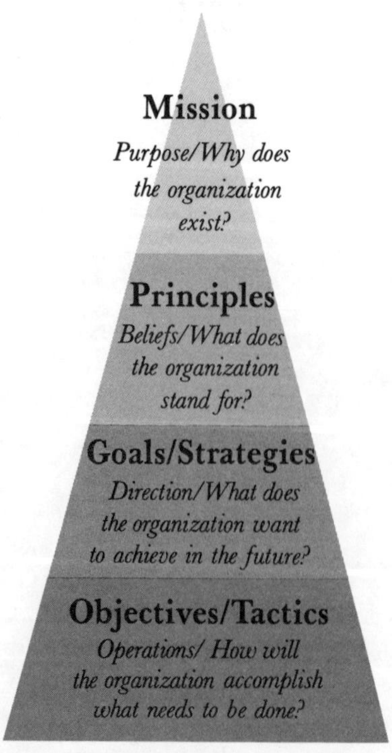

FIGURE SIX:

An Example of How a Planned Parenthood Might Articulate the Top Two Levels of the Planning Pyramid: Mission and Principles

MISSION:
to further the right of every person freely to make voluntary, informed decisions about sexuality, reproduction, and parenting and to assure the opportunity to act upon these decisions. To achieve this mission, we will promote, develop, and provide accessible and high quality services with special concerns for under-served, low-income, adolescent and minority populations.*

** The mission statement of Planned Parenthood of Northern New England*

PRINCIPLES OF PLANNED PARENTHOOD**

*** Author's statement of principles or beliefs*

1. stands for choice and must ensure that in each and every community, all choices can be exercised even by the young and poor, and even if this means we provide the means ourselves;
2. believes that all people, including children and youth, have a right to be knowledgeable about their sexual choices and learn how to behave responsibly, guided by their own individual standards of morality;
3. believes that its services must be universally available, especially to the young and the poor who might not receive those services if we did not provide or advocate for them;
4. believes that in spite of difficulties, we play three important roles—as health care and service providers, as advocates and as educators—and the synergy of these three endeavors multiplies our impact and makes us unique;
5. understands that our struggles are also about forging the popular consensus and political conviction necessary to garner the resources and programs for ultimate victory;
6. believes in being a stubborn and unrelenting champion of prevention first, intervention second, and purposeful intention always;
7. believes that there are no easy ways to reduce unintended pregnancy and premature parenthood, and therefore supports program innovation and new technology in order to solve these problems;
8. believes that the survival of this planet depends on creating a world where women and men can manage their fertility with safety and dignity and in concert with their own cultural and religious backgrounds.

GOALS/STRATEGIES: *To be arrived at by the board and senior management in their strategic planning work sessions.*
OBJECTIVES/TACTICS: *To be created by staff in order to achieve the goals, follow the principles, and remain true to the mission.*

responsibilities as one moves down the pyramid and ends up with a virtually exclusive domain in the *objectives/tactics* layer, where business, financing, and marketing tactics are created. The *goals/strategies* layer has the most interaction between board and management. Here the organization makes the critical decisions about what are the right things to do in order to establish strategic direction into the future.

For purposes of illustration, Figure Six (on page 41) gives an example of filling-in-the-blanks of the top two layers of the pyramid. This is not meant to suggest that this is the only way to articulate Planned Parenthood mission and beliefs. But in my experience in doing planning with affiliate boards, we almost always end up with mission and belief statements very similar to these examples. My hope is that this illustration provides a starting point for the planning process and allows the board to move to the heart of successful planning—goals and strategies—as quickly as possible.

Conclusion. The lack-of-time-to-plan dilemma is grounded in reality, but the fact is that boards are already investing time, reacting to crises that often could have been mitigated by planning. If time is that tight, boards can use one of the simpler planning models. Often, a quick and dirty plan is eminently more helpful than elegant intentions to create the ultimate plan next year. Boards can also spread planning exercises out throughout the board calendar, so everything doesn't have to happen in two months before the next recertification visit.

In summation, the essence of long-range strategic planning by boards is as follows:

- Get beyond the present
- Strive for quantum leaps forward
- Use the board for mission control
- Borrow ideas from the very best plans
- Board planning cannot be reduced to grids
- Use the plan until it's dog-eared
- Plan with a pyramid

With these principles in mind, the board can create a visionary document and process.

Let's now look at the Planned Parenthood affiliate in Kalamazoo, Michigan, whose board literally planned its way out of disaster.

Planned Parenthood in Kalamazoo

THE INFRASTRUCTURE OF A PLAN OUTLASTS THE BUILDING

Setting the Scene. Planned Parenthood in Kalamazoo, Michigan, is an affiliate with only one clinic site, but that clinic provides a sophisticated array of surgical services, including abortion procedures. This is also an affiliate that operates in a conservative and reactionary state, where the state legislature has been firmly anti-choice for decades. This is a story that reminds Planned Parenthood of one of its worst nightmares (sudden violence) and of its earliest beginnings (a group of community citizens concerned about the cause of "every child a wanted child"). This is a story about how a board of directors rolled up its sleeves and did what was necessary to survive.

In One Night, Much Can Change.

Reproductive Health Care Center/Planned Parenthood of Kalamazoo, Michigan (RHCC/PP) was extraordinarily proud of its seven-year-old, 10,000-square-foot building, which contained a certified outpatient surgical facility and administrative offices. The beautiful state-of-the-art building was promoted in marketing programs and fund-raising appeals. In December of 1985, following a $350,000 capital campaign, the board ceremoniously burned the mortgage; in December of 1986, one year later, an arsonist burned the building to the ground.

In the ensuing months the affiliate had a new theme: "Planned Parenthood is *more* than a building." All subsequent events testified to the fact that someone *can* destroy a building, but no one can destroy the commitment that burns deeply inside a good board of directors. It is the courage and tenacity of the people—volunteers and staff—that makes the Planned Parenthood cause indestructible.

The arson, later deemed by federal agents as the "most sophisticated and costly of any clinic arson in the country," destroyed three-quarters of the building. The destruction was so dramatic, with a church "Choose Life" sign visible through the burned rafters, that PPFA used this photo in several magazine and newspaper ads. Ironically, the surgical suite, which was used for abortions (built behind state-mandated fire walls), survived with only water and smoke damage, while the remainder of the clinic and offices was completely destroyed. Kalamazoo had no federal, state, or United Way funding; it was financed by patient fees and private contributions. Thus, without services, there was no revenue. And with no water, electricity, heating, or security systems, services were not possible on site for 14 months. Ultimately, it cost 1.5 million dollars more to restore the building and equipment to pre-fire levels.

Fortunately, Kalamazoo had a strong tradition of board planning, earning high marks on this in recertification reviews. This attribute saved the day when the arsonist struck. Anticipating the possibility of a catastrophic emergency, Kalamazoo had previously made arrangements for alternative space in case of emergency. This was brilliant planning, especially for a one-clinic affiliate.

OBSERVATION: The best long-range planning deals squarely with the question: What is the worst that could happen? Boards that engage in this "worst case" technique of planning tend to have their priorities clearly in order. Every affiliate should ask itself: "Do I have contingencies to protect my area of biggest risk?" This approach forces hard choices, explicit judgments of what is most important and what is less essential.

When the Going Gets Tough. Louise Safron, the Kalamazoo executive director, remembers how the affiliate responded. "In retrospect, it is hard to imagine those first hectic days: no records, no desks, no equipment, no phones. Clients who had somehow missed the extensive press coverage arrived to find an icy driveway and a gutted building, not the pills, pelvic exam, or abortion they sought." Staff and board members took turns sitting in cars outside the burned building to reassure and refer clients. Within the first six hours, a working office was set up in the executive director's home, outfitted with computers, borrowed typewriters, and shoe boxes for files. For 12 weeks, this was home base. Medical, counseling, and education staff were housed, by prior contingency plan agreements, in excess space at three area nonprofit organizations. Three staff members were constantly on the road between the four sites as communication "runners."

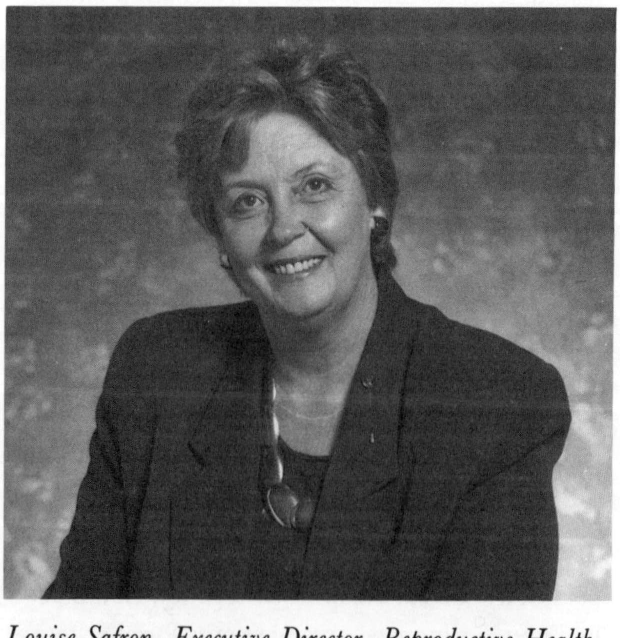

Louise Safron, Executive Director, Reproductive Health Care Center, Planned Parenthood of Kalamazoo, Michigan.

Board and Staff: Shoulder-to-Shoulder. One definition of crisis is an opportunity in disguise. Unfortunately, those "opportunities" arise very rapidly in an atmosphere in which decisions are demanded every minute without the usual luxury of time for gathering information and examining alternatives and consequences. Decisions on negotiating the insurance settlement, temporary quarters, guard service, new security systems, emergency fund-raising campaigns, and activities for reducing staff stress reactions all had to be made in a circus atmosphere interrupted constantly by media and the 24-member Bureau of Alcohol, Tobacco and Firearms team. In this atmosphere, the usual important lines between staff and board roles blur; thus, trust and respect among the board and staff become all-important.

OBSERVATION: The best test case for a strong board is a crisis. When an organization is stripped to its basic functions (by the loss of a key facility, loss of funding, or loss of an exceptional executive director), it returns to the essential core that gave rise to the organization in the first place—a committed group of volunteers now called the board. This responsibility to keep the mission going is the burden of ownership.

An Unusual Orientation: Trial by Fire. At the Kalamazoo affiliate, the board has defined four major responsibilities: hiring the executive director, setting policy, envisioning the future

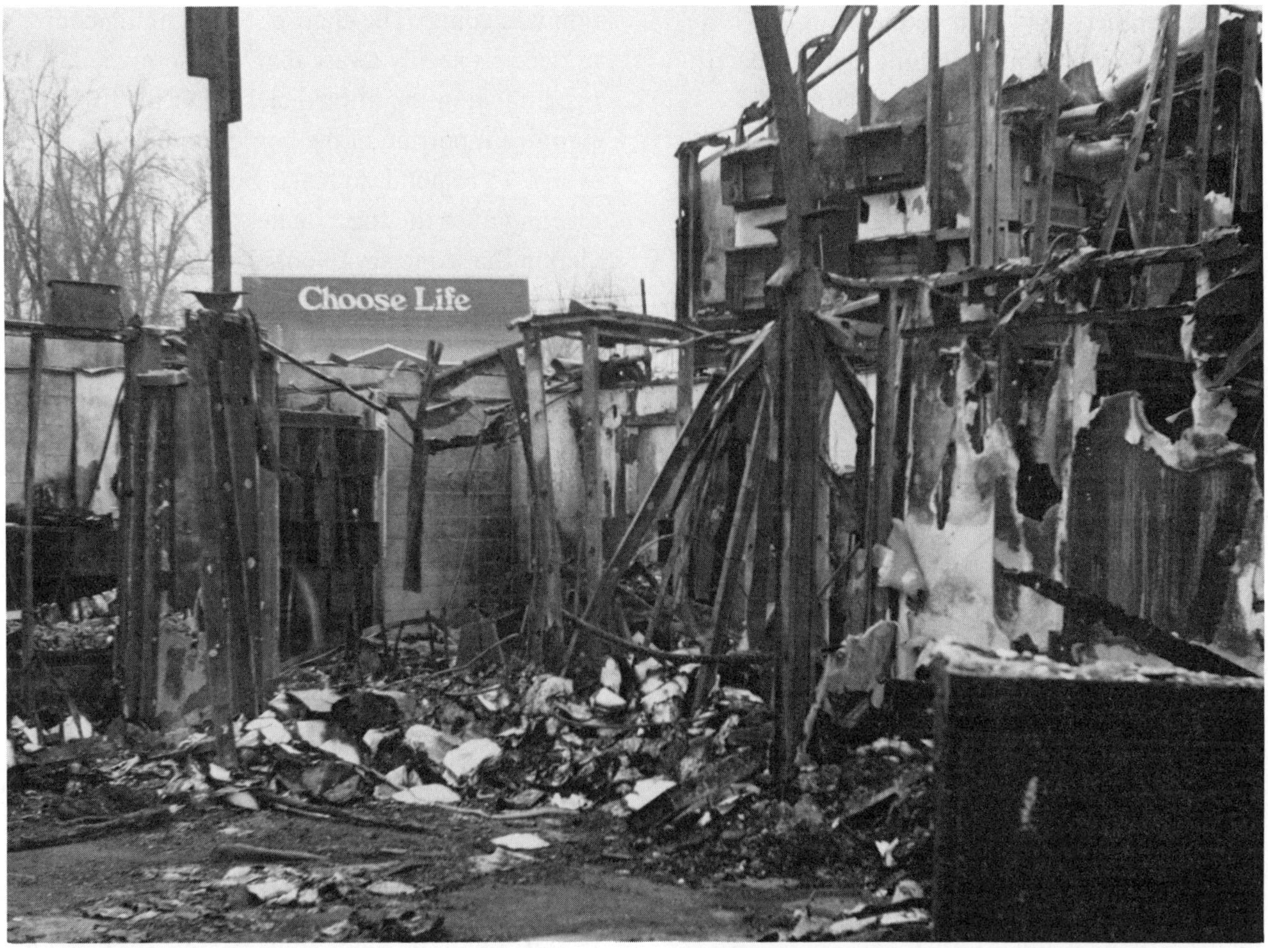

Arsonist torches the Kalamazoo Planned Parenthood clinic in December of 1986.

(planning), and ensuring the financial health of the organization. Many organizational textbooks state that the Nominating Committee is the most important committee of the board. This crisis proved that rule. One week before the catastrophic fire, four new board members had been elected and a new executive committee formed, all duly oriented. These four rookies already knew their roles and were willing to use their skills, contacts, and time to do what was needed. The nominating process had replenished the talent of the board and had given its newest members sufficient fuel so they could share in keeping the flame alive on some very cold winter nights in south central Michigan.

OBSERVATION: Boards must possess a healthy mix of members who can collectively have success at the three "W's" —Work, Wealth, and Wisdom. One of the time-honored truisms of people who make successful board members is that they have either the time and inclination for hard work, or the capacity to give/get generous donations from persons with wealth, or the conceptual thinking that generates wise policy and planning. One of these attributes gets a person on a board; two gets a person on a Planned Parenthood board; and three gets a person into heaven.

The Board Shows Its True Grit.

In general, board members who possess at least two of the classic three "W's" —Work, Wealth, and Wisdom—usually prove to be successful Planned Parenthood board members. In Kalamazoo, board members used their connections and worked the community with unyielding tenacity. Just nine days after the fire, the board had secured a temporary medical facility, enabling staff to move in. Board members begged and borrowed furniture and equipment from the storage areas of businesses, hospitals, and other nonprofits. Within a week, a Facilities Committee began planning for the new building, meeting with architects, contractors, and staff.

As a working board, the Kalamazoo trustees knew that the professional staff members were responsible for what the agency accomplished in programs. The board's level of respect and concern for staff was evident when the board decided that even though there was only $80,000 available in insurance coverage when the revenue flow was interrupted, there would be no staff layoffs. Board concern for staff was unwavering. In fact, one board member found a psychologist willing to provide counseling for no fee for any staff member wanting it. Needless to say, in the wake of all the unsettling trauma, several staff availed themselves of the opportunity.

In order to respond to the financial calamity, a President's Committee from the board was formed and created the Phoenix Fund Campaign, which raised $168,000 in emergency operating funds the first month alone. This was an affiliate which normally raised $90,000 per year. In the next 14 months, the affiliate raised nearly $750,000. While it is easier to raise money in a crisis, this level of achievement would have not been possible without the careful selection and orientation of board members to their responsibility for the financial health of the organization.

Plans Help Most When the Going Gets Tough. Few people *like* planning; most would rather just *do* than plan. Fortunately, however, one of the board's key jobs at Kalamazoo had always been to establish where the organization was going. The chair of the planning committee was keenly aware that with so many tasks needing attention immediately after the fire, a significant portion of the board wanted only to do things, to respond, to react. But at the first board meeting after the fire, she held firmly to her conviction that contrary to popular opinion, these activities would be more effective if they sprang from a board plan. It was true that many things were happening at once, that there were early indications that the critically needed insurance settlement was being held up in dispute, and that the Bureau of Alcohol, Tobacco and Firearms appeared to be investigating the affiliate in response to an anti-abortionist's charge that the affiliate had burned the building. Nevertheless, the planning chair handed the board a forced-choice planning exercise and requested that each board member spend 10 minutes putting actions needing attention in priority order. Never was mutiny so near. The action-oriented business men grouped in one corner and muttered. No one wanted to spend the time on this task *now.* Weren't there too many things to do? Respect for the power of planning—and the chair's tenacity—prevailed, and within 10 days of the fire, the affiliate had a one-page, 10-point list of short-term priorities for the crisis year. And in retrospect, the executive director believes without a shred of doubt that no one factor was more important to the recovery over the next hectic year as having had the board speak its planning conviction at the earliest possible point.

A Crisis Infrastructure Created. In a crisis, it is natural that the board will become more involved in affiliate operations and that it usually needs to create a temporary, short-term structure to deal with the increased work load. At Kalamazoo, the newly elected board president had been out of town on a trip when the building was torched. She returned to discover 14 messages on her answering machine about the arson. She immediately reorganized her calendar and went quietly to work organizing new committees to deal with the crisis and to use the energies of donors who "wanted to do something to help." She became responsible not only for the short-term success of finding gratifying work for the affiliate's volunteer supporters, but for a long-term change in the affiliate's mind-set about the use of volunteers in all capacities. Before the fire, the affiliate had only an occasional service volunteer, but since then, it has more than 35 service volunteers (equivalent of two full-time employees) and community volunteers serving on every standing committee. This proves both that necessity is the mother of invention and that the board leader knew to move back into the policy role when the emergency receded. Namely, she saw the extraordinary response of volunteers willing to help in desperate times and turned that into a long-term strategic opportunity for the affiliate to expand its human resources.

OBSERVATION: In stormy seas, use the strategic plan as a ballast and a tiller, not an anchor. Plans should steer and keep an affiliate in balance, rather than simply lock things into place. And since planning is more a process than a product, an emergent situation doesn't necessarily mean changing course—but it almost certainly means re-visiting the plan to see if core assumptions have shifted or to put broad principles into accelerated action.

The financial security of the organization had always been the fourth board responsibility at the Kalamazoo affiliate. After the fire, the fund-raising committees, with little or no staff direction, swung into gear with a three-part strategy: special events, large-dollar gifts, and donated materials. Sixty-eight days after the fire, 700 people gathered for an annual fund-raising event. The President's Committee rebuilt the 1,800 donor list, raised $168,000 in the first month, and secured $45,000 from each of the three major foundations in Kalamazoo. With donated equipment and supplies from businesses, hospitals, and other agencies, Kalamazoo was able to operate a 5,000-square-foot temporary facility with no major purchases.

OBSERVATION: There's gold in them there crises. Some charitable organizations pay expensive direct-mail copywriters lots of money to create the impression with prospective donors that indeed the "sky is falling" on that agency's cause. When real calamity strikes, boards can use it to break down long-standing fund-raising impediments. Reluctant solicitors are energized; the fund-raising case is being made on the front pages of the local papers; and any doubt about whether the affiliate needs the money is put to rest.

Looking Back. The destruction of a facility in a single-site affiliate is a dreadful, chaotic experience. It requires the board to rally in a rather extraordinary manner, as evidenced in the story of Planned Parenthood of Kalamazoo. If the board is a group accustomed to planning, it can fall back on that planning instinct. And if the board is a group used to private fund-raising, it need not flounder wondering what to do, but rather it can ask "how much?" and "when?"

CHAPTER FIVE:

THE BOARD AS POLICY SETTER

What Is Policy, Anyway? Policy may be the word most used and least understood by persons in nonprofit organizations. *Webster's New Dictionary and Thesaurus* defines "policy" as a "course of action adopted by an organization to influence subsequent decisions and actions." Policies are chosen by the board as the representatives of the general public, and they are chosen because they are believed to be sound and advantageous for the nonprofit organization. **Board policy consists of principles and procedures established to guide staff, to influence current operations, and to have an impact on the organization's future course of action.**

"The board makes the value judgments; management takes action."

MARGARET KANTNER
United Way Trainer

For example, let's say that the board believes that the organization and its constituents will benefit from a racially and culturally diverse work force. To manifest this value, the board ratifies policies of equal employment opportunity and affirmative action. These policies in turn require staff to search aggressively for qualified minority candidates, to consider offering English as a Second Language continuing education classes for new staff, and to report new hires and promotions in such a way that the percentage of minority staff can be measured.

Policy is best seen as referring to the broad, overarching, guiding principles to be used to make detailed and exacting decisions. It is both objective and subjective. It reflects core institutional values. Board policy represents the interests of the organization's stake holders—funders, patients, staff. Ideally, it gives management broad but clear guidance so the executive director can act with the security that the board has established a basic framework for programs, services, and management matters. Given this general direction, the executive director does not need to keep bringing operational issues back to the board. Board policies are an organization's constitution, and when assembled with the Articles of Incorporation and Bylaws, they provide guidance on how to run the organization in a prudent and expedient manner.

Every organization that has been in business for more than a couple of months has policies of some sort, even if they are informal. The organizational need to describe "how we do it here" is universal. To be most effective, policies need to be short, understandable, and sensible. They also need to be *written:* so that it is clear what they are; so that they will be remembered and used; and so that they won't be misinterpreted or used selectively.

Creating Usable Policies. My guess is that fewer than 10 percent of all nonprofits have usable, retrievable, future-anticipating policies that capture the board's values on matters of prudence, expedience, or other issues—policies that would give the organization an edge to succeed. Too often board policies are unorganized or inaccessible and, therefore, unusable. The lack of usable policies makes it difficult and time-consuming for the board to make decisions, because board members do not know what has been pronounced historically and must start from scratch. If policy is not stored and communicated properly, boards get themselves in the frustrating position of facing each new issue as if it had never been encountered before.

But if, on the other hand, the board has a written legacy from previous board deliberations, this can provide the foundation for consistent and coherent board oversight. A well-organized policy document keeps the board on track. It also becomes an obligatory part of board orientation for new members. It must be remembered that board membership is like a "relay race" in which individuals serve fixed terms and then hand off the responsibility to their successors. A good policy manual is like a baton, filled with the institutional memory and wisdom of 10 to 20 years of board deliberations and decisions.

The board must satisfy itself that it has articulated its intentions on every significant dimension of the affiliate. In other words, a policy must be established for every aspect of the organization in which the

> ***"For an institution, the continuity of trustees can be extremely important. Having an institutional memory has great significance. In some organizations, the learning curve can be complex and long."***
>
> **JEROLD PANAS**

board wants to provide overarching direction to staff. To many boards, this job seems overwhelming. But once done, it actually allows the board to stop worrying about the routines, minutiae, and rote habits of organizational process.

Let's take an example in an area in which the boundaries of policy and practice are particularly confusing—the revision of the annual budget. Affiliate budgets are highly dynamic in the '90s and can fluctuate dramatically within a single fiscal year. The question is this: When can the executive director independently make adjustments, and when does he or she need to return to the board for approval? In this situation, the board needs to determine what its policy will be when the current annual budget results differ from the board-approved budget. The board might decide that if any line item varies by more than 15 percent, a new budget is required. Or it might explicitly give the executive director the latitude to make adjustments based on new revenue forecasts, without needing to get board approval for a "revised" budget unless the bottom line moves into a deficit position. Either of these policies is fine—or a myriad of other possibilities could be crafted for a budget revision process. To determine what the policy should be for a particular affiliate, the board needs to weigh such factors as the overall agency financial condition, the executive director's performance in terms of financial management, and/or the expectations that funders have in terms of board involvement. The only wrong answer is for the board not to have a sound policy established, understood, and honored by all parties. The absence of policy in areas of importance can create confusion and resentment.

In a successful organization, often it is as important for a board to understand what it must ignore as it is to know what to attend to. For example, does the board intend to approve the individual items contained in the employee fringe benefit packages, or does it delegate that responsibility to the executive director? If it is the former, the board needs to make informed decisions. If it is the latter, the board needs to have some monitoring process to make sure that the executive director's judgments meet the terms of the policy that delegated this authority from the board to the executive director.

The Policy Manual. The repository of individual board policies should be a written manual. The manual should be organized by topic (e.g., finance, investment, conflict of interest, etc.). Every board member and senior management staff member should have a copy, should bring it to all board meetings, and should consult it when in doubt. The manual needs ongoing maintenance to reflect changes in policy and a thorough revision every other year.

The manual acts in some ways like a rulebook. The first priority is to address those areas in which the board wants to assert a value—e.g., all Planned Parenthood services shall be confidential and respect the privacy rights of all patients. Sometimes a policy needs to be very explicit because it attempts to balance countervailing forces—e.g., policy might state that the board seeks an optimum return-of-investment on affiliate fund reserves, but only if the investment portfolio is consistent with the Sullivan Principles (guidelines limiting investing in South Africa). In general, however, it is advisable to keep the policies broad enough so that they don't begin to resemble the kind of minute, nit-picking regulations for which governmental bureaucracies are famous. Four-inch-thick policy manuals are inevitably too detailed. Such precise regulations smother staff and invite loophole-seeking and adversarial skirmishes between board and staff. Good policies are to create trust, not to tear it down.

A Case Example of an Affiliate's Policy Manual. Abstract generalizations about what policy should or shouldn't do are sometimes too difficult to translate into practical situations. To remedy this in part, I felt it would be useful to provide a case study to show how one affiliate board, the board of Planned Parenthood of Northern New England, has drafted board policy for its manual. Because PPNNE is my own affiliate, it is the one I know best and can best use to illustrate points. Obviously, however, the policies described here are intended only as examples of how the board of one affiliate views its job of policy-making in issues important to itself and its chief executive officer. These policies spring from that organization's collective board values, culture, and style, and are not universally applicable to all affiliates. The PPNNE Board Policy Manual is organized around 10 key areas of affiliate life. The remainder of this chapter provides samples of policy in those 10 areas, each followed by a discussion that amplifies the rationale behind the policy statement.

PPNNE's 37-page board policy manual categorizes policy into 10 sections (see figure seven).

The board of Planned Parenthood of Northern New England has inserted itself in governing the operations of the agency only to the extent and depth that it feels necessary to fulfill its fiduciary, moral, ethical, and leadership responsibilities. It does so with pro-active policies and explicit limitations, rather than case-by-case judgment calls based on hindsight, which could appear to be second-guessing the executive director.

FIGURE SEVEN:

Planned Parenthood of Northern New England's Board Policy Manual

1. Mechanics of Board Operation
2. Relationship to the Public
3. Authority Delegation to the C.E.O.
4. General Statement of Values
5. Governing Style of the Board
6. Planning: Strategic and Operational
7. Financial Policies, Constraints and Prohibitions
8. Personnel and Human Resources
9. Monitoring and Assuring C.E.O. Performance
10. Philanthropic Funding

The board is not unaware of or uninvolved in operational activities; affiliate donors, grantees, and the public would find that irresponsible. But rather than spending precious meeting time reviewing the day-to-day operations, the board sets policies and then monitors on a sampling basis. This practice allows operations to absorb only 15 percent to 20 percent of board time and energy rather than the 80 percent to 95 percent one encounters on too many nonprofit boards.

SAMPLE #1:

MECHANICS OF BOARD POLICY: Governing Overview. The board is the fundamental governing body of the Agency. It serves as a link between the constituency and the C.E.O. Based on its set of values, it identifies tomorrow's needs and identifies services to be performed. It guides current actions through explicit policies. The board vests full authority in the C.E.O. to be responsible for managing the organization and carrying out board policies. Delegation of authority to the C.E.O. is of the "go until we say stop" rather than the "stop until we say go" variety. That is, having set out its vision and delineated what the C.E.O. cannot do, the board lets the C.E.O. manage.

The board makes decisions as a total body. No committee, including the executive committee, has authority to take action on the board's behalf unless specifically stated in the bylaws or board policies. The executive committee, as noted in the bylaws, is charged to act on behalf of the board in emergency situations or when a decision or authorization is required before the board is scheduled to meet as a whole. Committees or Task Forces may bring information to the board for attention and action. Ideally, this information is presented as alternative courses of action with the consequences analyzed. Board decisions are reached by majority vote of all board members acting as individuals.

Discussion. In the above policy statement on "Mechanics of Board Operations," the PPNNE board makes several things perfectly clear:

- *only* the board governs (not committees, not individuals);
- the board acts as the public's representative to its C.E.O.;
- its work is primarily anticipatory, not reactive;
- the C.E.O. manages the organization;
- the C.E.O. has complete authority if no board policy exists;
- committees are advised, when possible, to bring multiple options to the board.

Some might argue that this statement merely restates the obvious, but we have all watched organizations choke in "role ambiguity" between the board and the executive director. Thus, the articulation of precise policies can be essential, especially when trouble arises. There are still too many stories of development chairs who order fund-raising staff to make 32 changes in the spring renewal letter, or executive directors who are forced to pass up exciting new opportunities because the organization had no policy.

SAMPLE #2:

RELATIONSHIP TO THE PUBLIC: The Interdependent Relationship between PPNNE and PPFA. As an affiliate of a national organization we must abide by the policies and standards of PPFA. Thus, even though we are an autonomous, nonprofit corporation, to be affiliated with Planned Parenthood, we must operate within the framework of the obligations of the national 'trademark,' pay our fair share dues to remain an affiliate in good standing, and actively participate as a member organization in the deliberations and corporate decision making of our regional and national structures. It is our duty and responsibility to attempt to influence our national organization to adopt directives that are consistent with our affiliate's own perspective, the needs of our communities, and the articulation of local circumstances requiring national attention.

Discussion. This policy defines the "gate-keeping" relationship of an affiliate and the national organization. Sometimes it has been confusing and frustrating to figure out what it means simultaneously to be autonomous and to be bound to the dictates of the national organization. In this policy, the affiliate acknowledges that there are freedoms that we "trade off" in order to be part of a bigger federation; but at the same time, the policy makes the strong assertion that the board will be active in attempting to have the national organization do the right thing for the interests of local communities.

SAMPLE #3:

AUTHORITY DELEGATION TO C.E.O: Other Staff Members. The executive director is responsible to the board acting as a whole and is the only staff member so responsible. In the spirit of role delineation, the board should not direct any other staff member or attempt to resolve any staff issue, problem, or program with any staff member other than the executive director.

Discussion. No action may be more fraught with danger than when

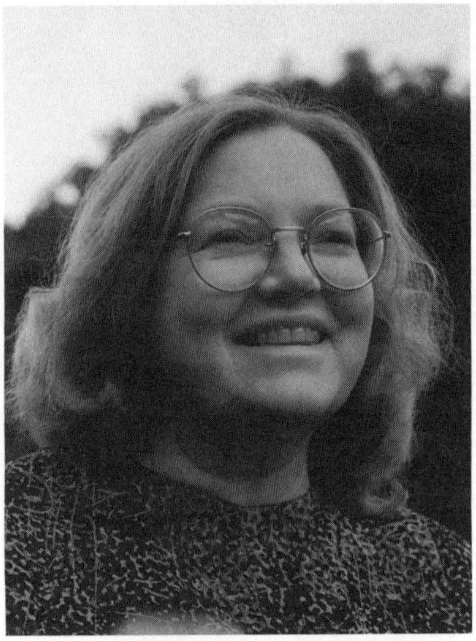

"Yes, boards should focus on the big ideological issues, but I believe that values such as business efficiency are also board concerns. Why? Because tolerating the wasting of time and money is a fundamental resources allocation question and that is board work!"

NORAH HOLMGREN

a board member attempts to troubleshoot, intervene, or problem-solve a staff issue. This policy makes it clear: If a board member wants to take up a matter involving staff responsibilities, he or she has one option: go to the executive director. This is not a gag order, because all organizations recognize the need for good communication between board and all staff members. But if the communication starts to become "supervisory" (e.g., give direction or solve disputes), the board member needs to cease and desist.

SAMPLE #4:
GENERAL STATEMENT OF VALUES: Effectiveness.
PPNNE shall provide its services and conduct its business in a cost effective manner, avoiding bureaucratic, money-wasting, and time-wasting practices.

Discussion. Policies need not be only about mission issues, governance practices, and role delineation. Here, the affiliate board wanted to be explicit: optimal effectiveness is expected, cost efficiency is sought, and waste of time and money is to be avoided. Thus, when the C.E.O. presents a budget or discusses productivity measures or faces the necessity of staff cuts and retrenchment, he or she need not worry excessively what the board will think—even if it is some board member's favorite program!

SAMPLE #5:
GOVERNING STYLE OF THE BOARD: Board Member's Code of Conduct.

- Directors must be loyal to the interests of the organization and constituency.
- Members have a responsibility to withdraw from decision making in cases of conflicting loyalty to outside advocacy or interest groups and membership on other boards or staffs.
- This accountability supersedes the personal interest of any director acting as an individual consumer of this Agency's services.

Discussion. Board members act as the group that sets the standards for the ethical behavior of the organization. Because of this, they must lead by example. This "code of conduct" policy frames the values of loyalty to interests of clients and then of the organization. Acknowledging that board members naturally will be involved with other often-kindred organizations, the code requires that if divided loyalties might be perceived in any issue to come before the Planned

Parenthood board, board members are obligated to excuse themselves from voting on that matter.

SAMPLE #6:
PLANNING: STRATEGIC AND OPERATIONAL: Annual Budget and Plan. The executive director must operate within a board approved annual budget of revenue and expenditures, with a separate capital equipment budget. The annual budget, prepared by staff, will be based upon the reporting of the past year's accomplishments, will track the progress of strategic initiatives and will be accompanied by a narrative of yearly objectives.

Discussion. The board explicitly states what information it requires when faced with the budget decision. Once the budget is approved, the C.E.O. is expected to operate within that budget. Subsequent policy statements (not quoted here) define the latitude that the C.E.O. has been given to revise and alter the budget and provide benchmark points at which the board itself would need to reconsider budget changes.

SAMPLE #7:
FINANCIAL POLICIES, CONSTRAINTS, PROHIBITIONS: Borrowing. PPNNE shall attempt to keep its debt load (both short- and long-term) at a conservative level. It shall not use debt-financing for operations, except in emergency situations or when a reasonable three- to five-year payback can be anticipated. It may also be used to level cash flow. If used for Plant Fund purposes, the following criteria must be met:

1. multiple alternative financing is explored, with decision based upon interest rates and flexibility;
2. internal financing via reserves has been rejected;
3. estimated property appreciation can reasonably be projected to recoup investment if the organization could not continue to carry the debt load.

No borrowing of funds is permitted unless it is consistent with a line of credit or indebtedness policy approved by the full board. No use of credit is permitted unless it is promptly reported to the budget and finance committee.

Discussion. In its financial borrowing, the board has determined that its principal financial responsibilities do not lie in detailed oversight of current operations. Staff take primary management of the monthly *income statements;* the board can then be liberated to focus on the *balance sheet.* Specific board attention is directed to reserves, investments, debt load, and contingencies for the future. This excuses the board from any nervousness about such relatively trivial concerns as to "why out-of-state travel is so high," and onto the long view considerations, such as, "Do we have enough money set aside to fund the clinic expansion?" In this subsection, the PPNNE board describes its philosophy on borrowing money:

- be conservative—do it sparingly;
- borrow to purchase assets, not subsidize operations;
- if borrowing for real estate, the most flexible mortgage is preferred; in fact, indebtedness is to be acquired only if the affiliate can't spare its own reserves and if the long-term investment prospects look good;
- report any use of pre-approved lines of credit to the budget and finance committee.

SAMPLE #8:

PERSONNEL AND HUMAN RESOURCES: Hiring/Promotion. Staff members shall be hired on the basis of abilities alone, without discrimination as to age, race, religion, gender, sexual orientation, national origin, marital status, socio-economic status, or disability. PPNNE is an equal opportunity employer. In the letter and spirit of its affirmative action plan, PPNNE will seek minority applicants for staff positions. Additionally, given PPNNE's services to women and large percentage of female staff, management and supervisory personnel positions will seek to provide opportunities for women in key management positions.

Discussion. The PPNNE board does not approve personnel policies; these are delegated to the executive director. Instead, it states its values related to issues of discrimination and its firmly held convictions on seeking minority job applicants and placing women in leadership staff positions. Keeping personnel policy and practice discussions (e.g., "How many vacation weeks should a second-year employee receive?") off the board agenda has freed up hours of board discussion time each year.

SAMPLE #9:

MONITORING AND ASSURING C.E.O. PERFORMANCE: Audit Presentation. The audit shall first be presented at a budget and finance committee meeting, with the audit firm in attendance and prepared to handle any inquiry or concern. At this meeting, there shall be a time where the staff is excused and the auditors will meet the budget and finance committee in executive session. Any significant findings discussed in the executive session will be shared with the executive director by the chair of the budget and finance committee. The yearly audit and the accompanying management letter shall be presented to the board at the next regular meeting following completion of the audit for their review and response. Any board member shall be allowed to ask for the auditor to attend such a meeting.

Discussion. In the above section, a protocol is established in order for the board to benefit from the tens of thousands of dollars spent each year on financial audits. The board gives itself permission to look as closely as it needs to and to talk directly with the C.P.A.s who have spent weeks reviewing the financial condition and practices of the affiliate. In and of itself, this may seem like overkill, but at PPNNE, having confidence in, and detailed knowledge of, the audit and what it means allows the board to spend significantly less time reviewing ongoing financial operations.

SAMPLE #10:

PHILANTHROPIC FUNDING: Confidentiality of Mailing Lists. Master lists shall not be given, loaned, or rented to other organizations without the approval of the board of directors. The confidentiality of our anonymous givers will be protected under all circumstances. The mailing list shall not be made available to political candidates for either information or fund-raising purposes. Donors who give explicit permission for the use of their names may have their names listed in the Annual Report.

Discussion. This affiliate policy takes a very hard line in protecting the identification of donors. The policy asserts an affiliate value choice that it is more important to keep donors' names exclusively within the agency than to be in a position to share lists with kindred organizations. This is an ethical dilemma; there is no one right answer. In policy discussion of such a matter, a board gets to wrestle with some interesting and complex issues.

Creating a Process to Pull Together a Board Policy Manual.

If an affiliate has a sketchy, out-of-date, or non-existent repository for board policies, it is a big assignment to create a coherent, contemporary policy manual. Here are some suggestions that can make such a daunting task more manageable.

- Appoint a high-level task force (e.g., including former board presidents) to create or revitalize the policy manual.
- Designate a person (most likely, the executive director or a staff designee) to do the actual writing of the drafts.
- Determine those aspects of the organization needing formal board policies; each of these will become a section of the manual.
- Scour board minutes over the past 10 to 15 years and pull out all policy decisions or actions that implicitly suggested policy. (Some organizations have been shocked and disappointed to see how few policies they actually uncover.)
- Brainstorm "informal" policies: instances in which, by tradition or custom, the board has relied on "phantom policies," but the exact precedents for these cannot be located. Next, express these "phantoms" in writing.
- Review the policy manuals of other affiliates and the national office and adapt those policies to your affiliate, especially where you have a void or an unwieldy current practice.
- Take into account the legal fiduciary duties (e.g., care, loyalty, and obedience) of boards to make sure that they are covered in your policies. Legal counsel should review your drafts.
- Reserve a major block of time at several board meetings so that the board gets to discuss and thoroughly understand the policy manual before it is ratified.
- Assign to a standing committee the task of keeping policies fresh and relevant. Again, since this is a critical responsibility, it must go to a group containing a majority of board leaders. (Executive or planning committees have been used with success).

Conclusion. When PPNNE took on this task of developing a policy manual, we began virtually from scratch. The process took almost a dozen meetings of the policy-drafting group, and the "draft" manual became the subject of a board retreat held about 24 months after the process had begun. PPNNE liberally borrowed and traded policy ideas from two other affiliates (Planned Parenthood of the Rocky Mountains and of Metropolitan Washington) which were simultaneously creating more explicit governance policies. Although the job sometimes became tedious, the resulting policy manual has paid for itself several times over. The benefit of having written explicit policies is that it eliminates uncertainty and enables the board to anticipate organizational decisions so that it is clear who, what, when, how, and why the organization should proceed—on almost any particular manner.

CHAPTER SIX:

THE BOARD AS BOSS

Overview. The scale and scope of the executive director's job in Planned Parenthood changed dramatically in the 1980s. Affiliate budgets have doubled, and the ratio of earned income to grant income may have sextupled. Executive directors can no longer dabble in politics, but must master its intricacies. The C.E.O. also must deal with fierce competition—for service delivery, for fund-raising dollars, for the most talented staff. Executive directors of top notch affiliates must navigate two worlds: first, they must possess "cutting edge" management and leadership skills comparable to those found in private corporate America; and second, they must excel in the public sector, doing comprehensive tasks such as building coalitions to affect public policy and practicing the best in public health administration.

"At the same time, every nonprofit, except maybe the very small and purely local one, must also have an effective executive officer. Its success in this century has made the American nonprofit too big, too complex, too important to be managed by a board."

PETER DRUCKER

"Ah, the temptation is great—but keep your hands out of the operation! Trustees are not to manage the institution, but to make certain that it is managed well."

JEROLD PANAS

"It's your job to evaluate the chief executive officer on a regular basis, and provide appropriate compensation. If you have a particularly good person, by the way, there's no harm in having the highest paid in their classification. If they're really good, why not? Someone has to be the highest."

JEROLD PANAS

In trying to find the person to fill this demanding position, boards often have a difficult job attracting and retaining a first-rate executive director. Affiliates that suffer from this affliction are continuously behind the proverbial eight ball. Simply put, if the affiliate doesn't have the right executive director with the requisite skills, talent, and commitment, the board will do no better than cope.

In my survey with board presidents, in my interviews with board leaders, and in the organizational literature, I have found an overwhelming consensus that the abilities and talents of the executive director are among the most important assets of an organization. Unfortunately, boards often settle for the best executive they can find and afford, not necessarily the best person for the job. Typically, this happens because the salary, benefits, and working conditions are not good enough to make the position acceptable to the best pool of candidates. Some boards still are stuck in the era when working for Planned Parenthood was an act of charity and an implicit vow of poverty. Furthermore, too many affiliates are simply not large enough (i.e., do not possess an adequate level of financial resources) to afford what they need.

The very best boards understand that the executive director of a Planned Parenthood is the chief executive officer of a corporation that is complex and challenging, the operation of which requires considerable skill and imagination. Let me suggest that finding and keeping this kind of executive in 1992 requires a salary in the range of $60,000, or significantly higher, depending upon the size of the affiliate and cost-of-living factors. If an affiliate cannot afford this salary, then it probably will not get the kind of talent needed. There could be the good fortune of circumstances (e.g., the executive director in a two-income family might accept a lesser salary), but that is not something to count on. Rapid growth and expansion or a merger may be ways to afford a real star or to hold on to the one the organization already has.

This is not to suggest that the only issue is money when it comes to locating and holding onto a great executive director. Other pertinent issues addressed later in this chapter are the ways in which the board searches for, oversees, evaluates, and if necessary, terminates an executive director.

Oversight versus Supervision: The board as "boss" is a role more easily discussed than put into practice. The image of a boss conjures up the notion of one person who provides oversight to subordinates, helps develop work plans to carry out job duties, and coaches staff as to how to accomplish tasks to meet predetermined performance standards. This kind of boss does what a boss does by *supervising.*

But a board is not that kind of boss. The board observes the executive director in action quite infrequently. Most board members do not possess the technical expertise to give the C.E.O. corrective feedback or positive coaching. Furthermore, a board is too large to provide such supervision; boards of 25 members have the potential to think that any particular task could be done 25 different ways. And that is not the kind of direction the chief executive officer needs. If the C.E.O. needs to be "supervised" in order to be successful, then the board has not selected a person with sufficient experience, judgment, or expertise.

What should the board do as boss? *The board provides oversight and evaluates the progress of the corporation and holds its C.E.O. accountable for these organizational results.* If the affiliate board has ratified a long-range strategic plan and adopted a set of comprehensive policies, more than enough baseline information exists to examine at what level the C.E.O. is performing. Using this approach, the destiny of the affiliate and the executive director are inextricably linked.

In other words, if the organization is doing well (under the specific set of circumstances confronting the affiliate), then it must be presumed that the C.E.O. is doing well. Clearly, there are other monitoring reports that can be used to enrich and broaden the board oversight function. The most relevant examples are: the annual financial audit; PPFA recertification reviews; and PPFA indicators of patient growth rates, financial ratios, and productivity rankings.

Evaluating the Executive Director. Performance appraisal is difficult under the best of circumstances, but when the supervisor is a collective, a board of 15 to 40 individuals who serve part time and hold diverse views, the job can be overwhelming. With creativity and dedication, approaches can be created that work well. C.E.O. appraisal must be done carefully, because the C.E.O. deserves to know what is being done well and what must be improved. In simplest terms this is how an appraisal enables executive directors to get better: they can relax a bit in job areas that are perceived as excellent and focus their improvement plans on the weakest aspects of performance. Boards do not have to be able to teach or correct for performance deficiencies; for that, there are hundreds of workshops, college courses, training tapes, and publications. But the mandate is to focus attention on strengths, potentials, and problems, because if the board doesn't do it for the executive director, no one else will.

The chances that a board will do well in its role as evaluator of the executive director are greatly increased if the board has in place the foundations discussed in the last two chapters. Using the written plans

> ***"Many boards incorrectly regard evaluation as a negative process and are uncomfortable in attempting it. However, when the process is well planned and fair, and when board members bring both close attention and good will to it, everyone involved benefits."***
>
> **ANDREW SWANSON**

and policies that define the results, the acceptable means, and the agreed-upon bottom lines, the board has the benchmarks with which to appraise the performance of the affiliate C.E.O.

> ***"The issue of evaluation of Planned Parenthood affiliate Executive Directors is often anxiety-producing for both the Executive Director and the board members conducting the evaluation.***
>
> ***Why? In evaluating the various formats presently existing for evaluating Executive Directors, there appears to be an inordinate amount of attention to subjective criteria that board members often have little information on or simply "don't know." From the Executive Director's perspective the subjective criteria often lack precision and have less application to the day-to-day aspects of the job."***
>
> **From the PPFA Southern Region Council**
> ***Executive Director Evaluation Guide***

The following essential ingredients are prerequisites for the board in order to effectively evaluate its C.E.O.:

1. ASK THE EXECUTIVE DIRECTOR TO DO A SELF-EVALUATION. Appraisal starts with asking the C.E.O. to evaluate himself or herself. Encourage candor and offer assistance where weaknesses are acknowledged or problems identified. The format can be flexible, but some fairly open-ended questions can be helpful. Here are some possibilities:
   - What do I consider to be the important abilities that my job requires?
   - What are my major accomplishments for the past year?
   - How do my personal achievements compare with affiliate performance?
   - In what area of my job do I need to improve?
   - What are the ways in which the board can help me to do my job better?

- In what aspects of my job do I feel I need more experience and training?
- What have I done for my personal and/or professional development?

This self-evaluation report should be discussed at the actual performance review session.

2. USE OVERALL ORGANIZATION RESULTS AS A BENCHMARK. The performance of the organization (successes and failures) is not necessarily synonymous with that of the executive director, but they are interrelated. Therefore, the C.E.O. should be appraised simultaneously with or on the heels of a thorough evaluation of the affiliate's achievements. Every board should have the executive director (as part of an annual evaluation cycle) prepare a report on the actual performance results compared to the budget and planning predictions. Additionally, the actual results should be compared with the goals in the board's strategic, long-range plan. Documented results verify the progress of executive competence and become the basis for the board's trust in the C.E.O.

   Obviously, evaluation of the C.E.O. of an organization as complex and ever-changing as Planned Parenthood defies simple checklist type appraisals, whose answers are yes, no, or maybe. The analysis of results requires critical and sophisticated thinking. For instance, meeting a goal may connote executive competence or blind luck. The board needs to differentiate between a "windfall" or meeting a standard that was woefully low in the first place. Conversely, in certain circumstances, getting 75 percent of a goal may represent a minor miracle that could not have been pulled off without exemplary effort by the executive director. These are the judgments that the board-as-boss must make.

3. DO NOT INVOLVE OTHER STAFF IN EVALUATING THE EXECUTIVE DIRECTOR. Although staff members have direct knowledge about how the executive is doing, putting them in a formal evaluation loop is very awkward. This style of performance appraisal breaches the classic lines of authority and can thereby set a dangerous pattern of communication within the organization. The ability to obtain useful and dependable information is compromised because staff must constantly worry that their comments might get back to their boss. In addition, the context of staff comments is a result of many variables that the board simply won't know or fully appreciate. A knowledgeable and involved board can evaluate by

"Executive Directors are very sensitive to board members involving themselves in management issues. One of the concerns is that board members do not trust executive directors to manage. Board presidents, on the other hand, urged trust but wanted verification."

Excerpt from PPFA report, ***An Analysis of Executive Director Turnover in 1990***

itself, as long as it has a benchmark plan to measure executive accountability and policies that allow periodic monitoring of affiliate practices. A board must discern why its affiliate is doing well or badly and how the performance of the C.E.O. is affecting overall organizational performance.

4. ALLOW INVOLVEMENT FROM THE ENTIRE BOARD. A written checklist, with some opportunity for open-ended responses, allows even new board members to participate in executive appraisal. However, if members have no certain or direct knowledge in a specific area, they should be given the opportunity to defer judgment. The best evaluation documents I've come across were developed by the Southern Region of PPFA *(Executive Director Evaluation Guide)* and by Lee Minto *(Choosing an Effective Executive Director: A Guide for Affiliate Boards)*. Both contain forms used by the board to evaluate the C.E.O.

5. CREATE A SMALL, KNOWLEDGEABLE EVALUATION TEAM. This handful of board members should include the most experienced and capable people who have worked directly and closely with the executive. It should always include the board president. Along with the executive director's self-evaluation and overall organization evaluation tools, this team uses two data sources: their own direct observation of the executive and the collected responses of other board members. They must sort through and assimilate this scattered array of feedback so that it can be shaped into a fair and coherent critique.

6. PROVIDE A WRITTEN EVALUATION. This report should highlight the strengths and weaknesses of the executive, specify any improvements sought, propose possible training plans, and offer an overall conclusion as to how the executive director is doing. It should be provided to the executive in advance of the performance review session and should form the basis of the appraisal meeting between the team and executive. The executive director should be allowed to respond formally if major disagreement occurs. The results should then be reported to the board, in part or in whole, in executive session with the executive director present. At this meeting, questions or other comments from the board at large should be invited. The written evaluation is filed in the executive's personnel folder.

7. NEGOTIATE COMPENSATION SEPARATELY. It is important to conduct the appraisal first and the salary negotiation later. If the

two items are not separated, discussion of money will invariably dominate the appraisal interview, and important messages regarding performance may be lost. Clearly, the appraisal should be linked with the compensation, but they should definitely occur separately and sequentially. Many boards find it convenient and consistent to have the evaluation team also do the salary negotiation, as this job is unwieldy for the board as a whole. The compensation negotiating group must be knowledgeable about comparable salary rates and benefit packages, both in the local job market and within the Federation. Most successful boards do not ratify the exact terms of compensation, but rather delegate to the small group and subsequently receive a full report on the negotiation results in executive session.

> ***"Build security into your (C.E.O.) job with a contract that spells out what the board expects and insulates you from the negative whims of your board . . . multi-year contracts, renewable yearly, are an excellent way to insulate yourself from the uncertainty of board changes."***
>
> **DAN CAIN**

A Contractual Employee. Many executive directors operate with a written contract or letter of understanding between themselves and the board of directors. A contract can protect the interests of both parties. For the executive director, the primary benefit is stability. Namely, with a very difficult job and in an era of employment "at will," written provisions can offer protection. For the board, the most attractive reason is both stability and continuity. Namely, the board as boss is by definition a revolving group (the negotiating group of two years ago may be composed of entirely different persons in the present), so keeping things explicitly clear and written is essential.

The following terms and condition topics are the elements that are most frequently found in employment contracts:

- the period of time covered by the contract, with specific dates set for the next evaluation and compensation negotiations;
- salary and benefits defined, especially if certain items vary with agency-wide personnel practices or salary ranges;
- explicit definition of any special "perquisites" that the board has provided—e.g., company car, performance bonus, tax sheltered annuities;

> *"Performance appraisal is an opportunity for coaching and growth."*
>
> VAUGHN KELLER

- any special provisions or protections that will come into place at the time the executive director leaves the organization. Although there may not be any affiliates with "golden parachute" clauses or "non-compete" post-employment agreements with their current executive directors, this is a phenomenon beginning to happen in some service-related professions. Some executive directors have significant severance awards built into their contracts and believe this creates a "safety valve" that deters affiliate boards from moving to terminate in a serendipitous or hasty manner.

The bottom line is that in any contract the board makes with the executive director, fair and ample *opportunity for success* must be provided and appropriate channels for candid job-related dialogue must be put in place. If these pledges are met, the board is not only being the boss, it is being a good boss.

Terminating the Executive Director. If hiring is the most important job, then firing is the hardest job. Anyone who has fired someone knows the emotional toll that it takes. It is difficult because it dredges up such emotions as fear, anxiety, and empathy, and is surrounded by such emotion-laden terms as failure, denial, and rejection.

But firing employees is a fact of life. It can't be done cavalierly because firing C.E.O.s threatens their livelihood and may damage their professional reputation. Additionally, with the executive director so visible atop the staff hierarchy, the firing is a major organizational event, with a high possibility of widespread institutional trauma. It must be done professionally and competently.

Several time-tested recommendations regarding the competent dismissal are:

- If credible evidence exists that the executive director has exhibited gross misconduct of duty, the board may find it advisable to immediately suspend or fire the executive director.
- A board should not move forward with a termination of the executive director without advice from affiliate legal counsel.
- A termination ideally should come only at the end of a process in which performance deficiencies have been identified in writing, adequate time for improvement has been given, and documentation exists that performance has not returned to an acceptable level.
- Being generous with 1) a reasonable financial settlement, 2) opportunities to resign, and 3) outplacement assistance is decent and humane, and it may also provide some legal protection.

Conversely, executive directors also should understand that ultimately they serve at the pleasure of their boards. This job is not a lifetime appointment. Having the top job at a Planned Parenthood is a very demanding career choice; thus, minimal satisfactory performance year in and year out may not be good enough. If security and safety are paramount concerns for an individual, the executive director's job at a Planned Parenthood is not the right one to accept.

Search and Selection of a New C.E.O. Several excellent resources exist for the affiliate needing to find a new executive director. As mentioned previously, Lee Minto has authored the standard document for undertaking the recruitment process, called *Choosing an Effective Executive Director: A Guide for Affiliate Boards.* At the end of Minto's guide book is an excellent monograph, titled "Replacing the Long-Term Executive Director," especially pertinent for the challenge of finding someone after an incumbent has been there for many years. Both of these documents are mandatory reading for the board with a C.E.O. vacancy. Additionally, some of the larger affiliates have hired search firms to assist them, either by "head hunting" prospective candidates or by providing counsel to the search committee as it undertakes this complex assignment. One element that adds a major degree of difficulty to the search process is that it needs to be undertaken without managerial staff support, for it would be inappropriate for the departing executive director to be heavily involved.

Some general advice may prove helpful. First, follow the literal meaning of the word "search." Make the search active and aggressive. Remember that in the old west, the search party didn't do its job through classified ads and job bulletins – it got itself dirty and tired by riding down some wrong trails and dead-end canyons. Second, don't overlook "in-house" candidates or, conversely, skip the search process because the heir-apparent seems inevitable. Third, know what the compensation norms are in the local executive director marketplace and in national PPFA circles. The PPFA Regional Office in San Francisco publishes salary averages for executive directors, broken out by tenure and size of affiliate. Fourth, exhaust the networks, both formal and informal, within the federation, talking to many people who could become potential candidates or who could lead you to potential candidates.

Conclusion. In sum, boards must find the very best person for the job of the executive director, must evaluate him or her fairly, must provide generous compensation, and, in general, must provide an employment environment that provides incentives so that they can hold onto their executive director.

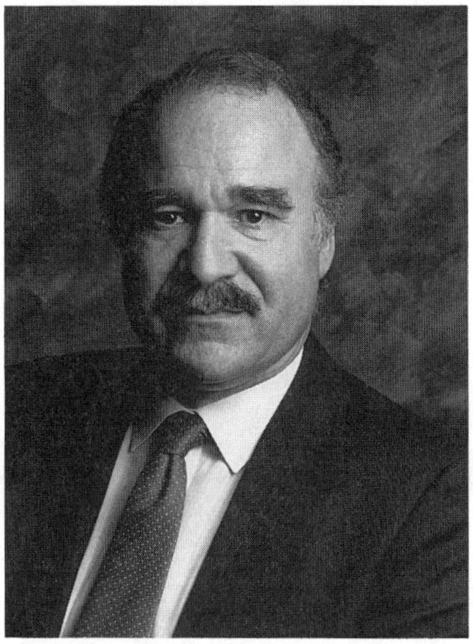

"There is no more important time for the board to assert itself than when the CEO leaves. The board must take the time to reevaluate and rethink what they want for executive leadership. It would be foolish to search for a clone of the past CEO. At first, the loss of the CEO is worrisome and anxiety provoking . . . but if handled wisely, it can be empowering for the entire board."

DR. KENNETH EDELIN
Former Chairperson PPFA Board

CHAPTER SEVEN:

THE BOARD AS FUND RAISER AND ADVOCATE

"Apart from the ballot box, philanthropy presents the one opportunity the individual has to express his meaningful choice over the direction in which our society will progress."

GEORGE G. KIRSTEIN

Money Raiser and Advocate: Are These The Board's Work?
Virtually all not-for-profit boards must plan strategically, set policy, and employ an executive director. At Planned Parenthood, these three basic jobs get expanded to include fund raiser and advocate. Board involvement in these additional activities is typically felt to be crucial because members often have contact with the influential opinion leaders who must be lobbied and with affluent members of the community who can finance our work with private donations. The assumption is that board members (rather than staff) are most likely to be peers of the movers and shakers in the community.

"The board provides proof to the community— especially in fund raising and public affairs— that the affiliate is grounded in what is good for the community."

SUE MOMEYER
Executive Director
Planned Parenthood
Association of Butler County

But I believe it is the two quotations from Margaret Sanger, on pages 70 and 76, that suggest most convincingly why fund raising and advocacy are board roles for Planned Parenthood affiliates and why I've chosen to cluster them together. Sanger knew all too well that although our movement could occasionally push back the curtains of sexual oppression and ignorance so that individuals could thrive, the forces of government and public policy would never behave properly unless we successfully engaged in the political domain. Sanger also knew that one doesn't raise money by simply sending out a memorandum that it should occur. People give money to people and they give more money to people who are working hard. It is not coincidental that the best fund-raising affiliates in the federation are also the most visible, committed public affairs affiliates. The varying levels of success in the organizations correspond directly to the degree of involvement by the board of directors. In other words, if the board works hard in fund raising, the affiliates raise lots of private dollars; if the board is only minimally involved, the affiliate probably raises way below its potential.

One of the reasons why many nonprofits don't involve their boards adequately in fund raising and advocacy is that since the board's *overall* responsibilities are so broad and vague, enough time is never left over for advocacy and fund raising. Furthermore, many charitable causes are so accepted by mainstream society that legislative mischief is unthinkable, taxpayer money flows freely, and board involvement seems almost gratuitous.

Another reason why some nonprofits don't involve their boards in fund raising and advocacy is that conflicts or stress between board and staff inevitably arise. Board involvement in lobbying and fund raising does not eliminate the need for staff involvement. Rather, these two functions become areas of shared responsibility. A certain amount of role ambiguity is inevitable when staff acts as both the supervisor (planning the tasks, making the assignments, checking up on results) and the subordinate to the board (staff work for the executive director, who works for the board). One clarifying approach used by many affiliates is to have the advocacy and fund-raising tasks separated, with staff working on the broad public constituencies (the mass), and the board focusing on the people whose contributions or influence can make a sizable impact (the class). This separation by target audience helps avoid confusion. Thus, the staff may be most involved in direct-mail and grassroots lobbying appeals. The board may be most involved in personally soliciting the affiliate's largest donors and getting to the chair of the legislature's appropriations committee right before a big budget vote on the family planning bill. Good boards and good staffs realize that working together on the same endeavors works only if individuals are primarily self-managed, if they don't require an over-the-shoulder supervisor, and if they do the work required of them in a timely fashion.

"Every experienced campaigner knows that money follows hard work. It is not the other way around."

MARGARET SANGER

The Board Fund-Raising Role

The Board Is a Peer of the Donating Public. Although donors contribute to Planned Parenthood because of their belief in our mission, the frequency and level of their giving is often influenced by who asks them for their gift. The fund-raising axiom that "people give to people" has been borne out in every campaign with which I have been associated. And because board members are not paid, they are unquestionably seen as the true believers, holding the most trust with many of our key donors. Good board members want to use their heads to provide wisdom on planning strategically, setting policy, and supervising the executive director. But to make the volunteer experience more complete and tangible, they may also want to roll up their sleeves and work. Board members are not trained to work with patients or to design the election year pro-choice media campaign, but they can find the crucial private dollars that underwrite key affiliate programs and undergird the institution's present and future financial security.

Some affiliate boards still treat fund raising as a dirty word and don't even triple their "fair share" dues amount (fair share historically relied heavily on wealth indicators in each affiliate's turf). In most of these cases, affiliates have not successfully engaged their boards in fund raising primarily because they have inadequate staff support or an inadequate structure to organize individual board members by matching their talents and experience with the tasks. But such affiliates are missing a great opportunity. In the next few pages, I suggest some efficient structures to organize the board and the necessary staff assistance.

"As a trustee, you do indeed carry responsibility for the 'extra margin.' These are the funds that transform a so-so organization into a good one. A good one into a great one."

JEROLD PANAS

Bad Times Beget Good Fund Raising. Fund raising at the affiliate level has generally improved, but the decade of the '90s promises to be even better. The irony in our field is that bad news in the public arena invariably translates to very good news for private fund raising. Thus, with a Supreme Court tearing away at privacy rights, with a federal government unfriendly to our work, and with the political action returned to our own state capitals, Planned Parenthood is in the fray, in the headlines, and in the hearts of our admiring donors—past, present, and future.

Meaningful, Substantial, Appropriate Board Involvement. It is easy for a board to nod yes when asked whether it does fund raising. If you've made one solicitation call or signed twenty letters, the board can indeed answer in the affirmative. But if the board opts for the minimum, the affiliate will not reap the harvest being gathered by the affiliates that make substantial fund raising a prerequisite for joining the board. Taking the lead in fund raising requires the board to spend a substantial amount of quality time, with focus on those areas in which sizable gains can be accomplished.

Does this mean that every board member is going to be equally involved and successful in fund raising? Of course not. Individual board members are blessed with different talents and varying degrees of access to wealthy individuals. What it does mean is that every member puts a *meaningful* amount of time into raising funds. In fact, this development duty should be in every board job description and a vital factor in every nominating decision.

There are many ways for boards to make good on this fund-raising responsibility. I'm not aware of any affiliates that have too many committed, hard-working, fund-raising volunteers. There are always potential donors needing solicitation; there are phonathons, envelope-stuffing parties, new lists of potential donors to be found; there are personal acquaintances and professional colleagues ready to be pitched. There is an old fund-raising bromide that boards must remember: "the money does not just walk in and surrender." What it takes is hard work at both the staff and board level.

FIGURE EIGHT:

Fund-Raising Tips

- Executive directors should be personally involved in targeting, cultivating, rating, and screening the top 10 percent of affiliate donors. They should also solicit or be part of a solicitation team to the affiliate's most important donors.
- The aggressive PPFA direct mail campaigns of the last 10 years leave every affiliate with the names of prospects, many of whom are anxious to get connected locally.
- The opportunities for special campaign efforts—e.g., endowment, capital, political—are many. Often these campaigns push affiliate fund raising quantum leaps forward by raising contributors' sights and making affiliates visible—especially bricks-and-mortar capital campaigns.

> ***"When we ask for money, we are friends, not adversaries. We are counselors, not salesmen. It's not a game of predator and prey. We are trying to help the donor do something significant for the community and for society."***
>
> **JAMES GREGORY LORD**

The final factor of note is that board members in most circumstances should exclusively focus their development work in *soliciting individuals for big gifts.* Soliciting is simply a big word for asking. And asking for money for Planned Parenthood is something that every board member can do. Fund raising is not an innate talent given to only a few; does not require a silver spoon or a stock portfolio; does not require a holiday card list of 200 society patrons; and does not require that one

> *"Remember the three 'G's: Give, Get, or Get off."*
>
> OLD BOARD ADAGE

possess a personality quirk that craves rejection. All it takes to be a good fund raiser is good training, good materials, and an opportunity to practice. This is the stuff that staff supplies. All that a board member needs to bring to the table is courage, conviction, and perspiration.

The Bedeviling Problem of Board Structure Geared to Fund Raising. A problem that many boards have is that the organizational structure is not geared to the development task, which is specialized and meaningful enough for the board as a whole to be involved. Thus, what often happens is that an overburdened development committee heroically tries to do everything possible and resorts to pleading and cajoling the remainder of the board when the end-of-the-year panic hits.

When confronted with this dilemma, many affiliates have turned to one of the most knowledgeable and respected fund-raising consultants in the federation, Doris Critz Yankee. Yankee has been the chief fund raiser at Planned Parenthood of New York City and Planned Parenthood of Chicago, a regional fund-raising consultant, and Vice President for Development at her alma mater. Yankee believes that the key to optimizing fund-raising potential is to make it one of the primary considerations of the board.

To organize the board's fund raising, Yankee has produced a design that is admittedly somewhat elaborate and takes a large board to implement fully—but is capable of creative adaptation by each particular affiliate. One of its strengths is that this model creates an authority and accountability structure and a vehicle broad enough to have a place for every board member. What follows is a description of the Yankee ideal.

The Yankee Model. Yankee builds from a traditional assumption that one of the major functions of a governing board is to ensure the financial health and stability of the organization. To achieve that end, it is essential that board members not only make personal financial commitments consistent with their ability to give, but also recognize their responsibility to seek adequate funding for the policies and programs of the affiliate. At the time of election to the board, members should be informed that participation in at least one aspect of the development program is expected.

In the Yankee model (illustrated in Figure Nine on the next page), the board is organized into six work groups: the development committee and its five subcommittees: major gifts, special gifts, general appeal, corporate and planned giving. The model resembles a daisy. This development committtee structure is superimposed on the regular board standing committee responsibilities. Thus, a board member would have

FIGURE NINE:

The Yankee Model: Fund-Raising Structure for Boards

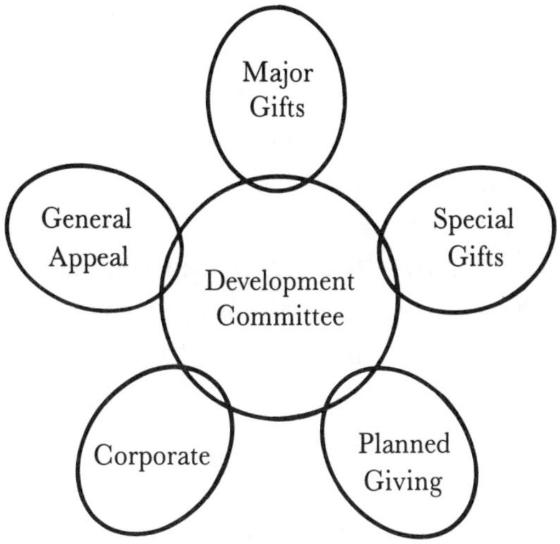

two committee assignments: on a regular standing committee and on a development committee. Here is the outline of the goals and duty assignments in this model. The suggested number of board members is based on a board of approximately 40 members.

The Development Committee as the Hub. The development committee, with appropriate support and guidance from the staff, should take the leadership and responsibility for meeting the financial needs of the agency through providing maximum support from the private sector. This group should consist of a chairperson, the chairpersons of all sub-committees for fund raising, two members-at-large from the board, and the president of the board. Its functions are: (1) to analyze past fund-raising programs and performance, search for meaningful trends, and identify strengths and weaknesses; (2) to adopt and coordinate an overall annual development plan for the affiliate; (3) to involve all members of the board in some aspect of fund raising, and to identify and attract to the affiliate others in the community whose work and support are needed; (4) to meet regularly to review fund-raising progress and develop strategies to increase private funding and identify new sources of income; and (5) to report regularly to the board on the fund-raising program.

> *"Board members should not only be involved in securing funds, but should also be integrally involved in determining how much money can be raised and how it should be raised."*
>
> **IRWIN STOOLMACHER**
> **Organizational Consultant**

Major Gifts Subcommittee is responsible for donors capable of giving $1,000 or more annually through face-to-face solicitation. It should

"The board's financial responsibility is development of financial resources—in other words, not just counting the beans but also in finding them and a garden to plant them in."

ANONYMOUS

consist of a chairperson, six to eight members of the board, past board members, and volunteers identified as experienced solicitors. Its functions are: (1) to assist in the identification of past and potential donors capable of making gifts of $1,000 or more; (2) to work with development staff in the training of volunteers in the techniques of personal solicitation and in making appropriate assignments of prospects to solicitors; (3) to undertake cultivation and solicitation of large donors and prospects; and (4) to help organize and participate in special cultivation events in private homes and in local clinics.

Special Gifts Subcommittee is responsible for the solicitation of gifts in the $500-$999 range through various forms of personal solicitation. It should consist of six board members and key volunteers from different sectors of the community. Its functions are: (1) to identify donors in the special gifts range and make personal contact through interviews, preferably, but at least through personal letters and telephone follow-up; (2) to personalize letters to donors and potential donors who are within shooting distance of specials ($100-$499); and (3) to help organize and participate in special cultivation events in private homes and clinic sites.

Subcommittee for the General Appeal assists staff in mailings to small donors (under $100), in organizing and recruiting volunteers for phonathons, and to assist in obtaining new lists to attract new donors. This subcommittee should consist of a chairperson from the board, four board members and additional volunteers recruited in outlying areas.

Corporate Subcommittee consists of a chairperson, preferably a prominent business leader, and three or four committee persons with good contacts in the corporate community. Its functions are: (1) to work with development staff in developing a list of corporations and businesses considered most likely to support Planned Parenthood; (2) to consult with other board members as to their corporate contacts or affiliations, and their willingness to participate in solicitations; (3) to identify corporate leaders willing to host luncheons or breakfasts for corporate officers on behalf of Planned Parenthood; and (4) to participate in the solicitation of past and potential corporate donors.

Planned Giving Subcommittee assists staff with a Planned Giving program. It should consist of board members, trust lawyers, and estate planners. Its functions are: (1) to determine what planned giving vehicles are appropriate (e.g., charitable remainder trusts, life insurance, etc.); (2) to advise on the development of a marketing strategy to targeted donors and targeted professionals (e.g., friendly tax-planning accountants, personal financial planners, bank trust officers); and (3) to set long-term goals in terms of solicitations and dollar-level goals.

In this model, each subcommittee chair will then hold an organizational meeting to adopt a goal and a timetable for the committee and to make assignments and explain procedures for reporting to the chair on a timely basis. Each subcommittee will need an appropriate development staff person assigned to provide staff support.

"It seems to me that the board must always 'keep its eye' on fund raising if it is to make responsible decisions, and it should be prepared to fulfill its financial role when making such decisions."

DORIS CRITZ YANKEE

Too much? Does this design proposed by Doris Yankee take more personpower and resources (e.g., time, energy, money) than most affiliates are willing and able to allocate? Probably yes. In fact, my biggest worry is that such a major fund-raising commitment could take the board's eye off its governance job if it is completely implemented. But this design is loaded with practical organizational ideas that can be taken in part and used immediately. For me, the Yankee model operates as a long-term ideal that our boards should constantly be reaching for and evolving towards.

Fund Raising Concluded (But It Never Is). Private development in a Planned Parenthood affiliate is a prime example of the 80/20 rule: in other words, 20 percent of the donors will produce 80 percent of the contributed income. Therefore, with so much riding on a rather select group of contributors, it is essential to provide them with "first class" treatment. This necessarily includes cultivation, communication, and solicitation in as personal a manner as possible. And what could make a better statement of key donors' importance than to have a board member as their link to the organization?

Let us end by observing the anonymous gardening analogy quoted on page 74. A board truly owns the trusteeship of the affiliate when its members contribute substantially to the development—both friend raising and fund raising—of the resources of the affiliate. Too many nonprofit boards fall into a passive monitoring, "bean-counting" style of governance when all the budget is produced somewhere else—like government. But if the board acts at its highest level—actively raising funds for clients and programs, it energizes its governance in a way similar to stockholders infusing their own hard-earned capital into a private company.

"Enlightenment will be extinguished . . . unless applied . . . to the machinery of political and legislative action."

MARGARET SANGER

The Board Advocacy Role

Again, the Volunteer as the True Believer. The board's ability to speak out as an unabashed believer in reproductive choice is more effective and convincing than any paid lobbyist can ever be. Staff can speak out and persuade, but often the board voice is many times more powerful. It is the volunteer's voice that translates Planned Parenthood's positions to our communities. The board leaders carry great reservoirs of credibility because they have no other vested interest except that of caring for the cause. Political, community, and opinion leaders often take their cue on our issues from the way board members articulate the position of Planned Parenthood.

Needing to Find a Structure. The missing element for many affiliates in terms of how the board can provide leadership in the public affairs arena has been how to do it. Because advocacy/public affairs is so radically different by virtue of the size and location of the affiliate, there is no single model to hold as a standard. But if the goal is to have the board provide oversight on advocacy and to participate actively as individuals in some public affairs task, each affiliate must create a structure that defines roles and tasks.

> *" Volunteers are rallying to our standard in the post-Webster environment, and their eagerness gives us a great opportunity to mobilize for victory. But wars are not won by the moving pageantry of people marching in the streets. Rather, the victories we need and seek stem from organizing clever, determined, and committed people with a clear vision of the results they must obtain into small, active, political units with well-defined, almost military, objectives.*
>
> *Simply putting names of fired-up volunteers on a public affairs mailing list is psychologically distancing; so is asking them to write an occasional letter. To help you make volunteering as*

satisfying as possible, we are offering a plan for organizing and activating volunteers to achieve important results, to enlarge the constituency of Planned Parenthood, and to do so in a manner calculated to meet each volunteer's personal need for action and involvement."

ANNE SAUNIER

Anne Saunier, who chaired the PPFA board from 1987 to 1989, wrote a paper about organizing volunteers for political success, *Organizing Volunteers to Get Results.* Although its focus was broader than just the board – i.e., volunteers as a collective whole – it offers recommendations that can be used by the board as advocate. As Doris Critz Yankee proposed a structure for fund raising, so Anne Saunier offers an explicit structure for a successful advocacy effort. A synopsis of Saunier's design is to organize the volunteer group (board or public affairs committee) into two teams: a *constituent* team and an *issues* team. The constituent team will focus on a key or problematic political official in order to gain the necessary clout or leverage to move that politician to vote in our interests; the issues team will become expert on the priority public policy items that have an impact upon our movement.

The constituent team is organized around the key elected political official in one's affiliate territory. The team undertakes the myriad of activities needed to become informed about and influential with their assigned politician. Team members might cross-match affiliate donors with political campaign contributions that went to the candidate; they canvass, organize petition drives, and register voters; they develop a vote-by-vote profile on the official; they visit the official and get the official to an affiliate's clinic; and they create "grass-roots" communication to pressure or thank the office holders for their supportive votes.

The issues team is organized around one discrete issue that is essential to the Planned Parenthood political agenda (e.g., federal family planning funding or state abortion rights). This team educates itself about its subject (e.g., its history, the process for enacting a law) and it helps collect the public policy materials needed to prevail.

Saunier then goes on to describe how these two efforts are coordinated through a matrix management approach. Whether every affiliate board wants to use this approach is really beside the point. The powerful notion at work here is that it is not enough for boards to have

"For an institution to grow and flourish it must be inherently vital, incessantly curious, aggressively courageous. Hungry for innovation, quick to respond to human need, willing to fight for a social agenda. Eager to face head-on challenges of the times."

JEROLD PANAS

"Look for board members in Planned Parenthood who like or can tolerate controversy."

ETHELYN BISHOP
Former President
Planned Parenthood of
Metropolitan Washington, D.C.

"good intentions" to be a powerful advocate. They must also possess an organizing scheme, with defined roles, with adequate time set aside to influence the public policy we care about and the public policy-makers who cast their votes.

Many Advocacy Roles from which the Board May Choose. It is in the realm of board members acting as individuals – but often representing the affiliate – where board members can become effective advocates. The options are many:

- lobby elected officials for support with the affiliate's public affairs agenda;
- represent the affiliate in a coalition for "choice" or health care reform or mandated sexuality education in the public schools;
- get training as a public speaker and address civic organizations to explain the work of the affiliate;
- provide testimony at a public legislative hearing;
- register voters;
- get involved (as a private citizen) in party politics so that one gets to know the cast of characters and become a player.

The bottom line is that every day and in every way, board members should prepare themselves by knowing the core principles of what Planned Parenthood stands for and should act as an advocate in the many different professional and social situations that are part of their lives.

Conclusion. In the last decade it has become abundantly clear that Planned Parenthood's success is closely linked with power and money. The modern-day reality is that it is simply no longer sufficient that our cause is just or that a majority of citizens support our programs. Planned Parenthood is in a fight for the heart and soul of the American public, and it takes political muscle and big bucks to prevail. Our opponents are well financed and often have church structures available to take the battle to us. For this reason, affiliate boards must find the right structures and must plan carefully to get the most from their public affairs and fund-raising efforts.

Planned Parenthood of Seattle-King County:

A BOARD FOR ALL SEASONS

Setting the Stage. Planned Parenthood of Seattle-King County (PPSKC) has been for many years one of our federation's strongest affiliates. Its boards have been particularly brilliant lights, whose collective actions have helped to create an exemplary organization and whose individuals have moved up through the ranks of regional and national boards. Yet several years ago, the affiliate's falling-out with its local United Way received national media attention. The affiliate's ultimate triumph has empowered local affiliates all throughout the country who have United Way funding. This is a story about a board that turned to its core beliefs to guide it through the turbulence, one whose executive director and board chair were role models of the ideal leadership partnership. This story also reaffirms the fund-raising truism that if a cause or organization is in real jeopardy, donors will respond generously.

Independence Threatened. The combination of a knowledgeable and involved board, talented staff, a supportive community in the largest metropolitan area in the state of Washington, and a vigilant free press, allowed Planned Parenthood of Seattle-King County to convert a financial crisis into a genuine opportunity for growth and independence.

For almost 20 years, there had been many nonprofit and proprietary abortion clinics in the Seattle service area providing high-quality and low-cost care. But during the mid-1980s, as the insurance and political climate worsened, these providers began to disappear. At that point, the PPSKC board responded to the new reality.

OBSERVATION: When the environment changes, affiliate initiatives must respond. Good strategic planning starts from a thorough scan of the external world, looking for threats and opportunities. And sometimes the ground shifts and the sea changes. The threat was that safe, affordable abortions for Seattle's patients were becoming hard to obtain; the opportunity was that this affiliate possessed all the prerequisites to expand into this service niche and to help patients meet a need.

Early in 1988, the Seattle board came to the unanimous decision to begin providing abortion services in order to protect access for its low and marginal income patients. Recognizing that the decision could be controversial, Seattle's executive director, Lee Minto, set up a meeting with the local United Way which was providing the affiliate with $447,000 of its $4,500,000 budget. She told them that the affiliate would not seek funds for the new abortion service, but only for existing education and family planning services that had historically been subsidized by United Way dollars.

Storm Clouds Gather. Initially, United Way said little about the new service. Other groups were not as quiet. The Catholic Church's

United Way ousts Planned Parenthood

By John Hessburg
P-I Reporter

United Way of King County, pinned between two adamant opponents in the argument over abortion, last night voted to oust the local Planned Parenthood group as a member agency.

Under a proposal approved by United Way directors, Seattle-King County Planned Parenthood would split into two separate agencies. One would be funded by United Way and would not offe[r] abortions. The other would get n[o] United Way funding and woul[d] provide abortions to a four-county area.

... non-abortion ... un- ...

against funding abortions or any agencies that perform them. But Planned Parenthood, one of United Way's member agencies, has [d]eclared it intends to offer abor[tions] ... County next year. ... [recomm]ended

Planned Parenthood says 'NO!' to United Way plan

By Mary Rothschild
P-I Reporter

Planned Parenthood of Seattle-King County yesterday decided to go without United Way funding rather than be forced to divide into two corporations in a dispute over abortion services.

"(We) will not reorganize to meet the demands of the Roman Catholic Church," said the family-planning group in a prepared statement released immediately after a closed-door board meeting.

The loss of United Way funding could amount to more than $400,000 – about 10 percent of the group's annual budget – which Planned Parenthood representatives said they will raise in an "appe...

> "We will not reorganize to meet the demands of the Roman Catholic Church
> – Statement of Planned Parenthood

community who endorse freed[om] of choice."

They vowed t... aggressive... the...

But during a news conference following the decision, Planned Parenthood board chairwoman Georgie Friedenberg and others repeatedly said their real quarrel is not with United Way. They blamed the Catholic Archdiocese of Seattle for stripping away Planned Parenthood's 18-year membership in the fund-rais[ing] agency.

"We are d... United W...

United Way campaign hurting

Dropping of Planned Parenthood leads to falloff in collections

By Gil Bailey
P-I Reporter

Top officials of United Way of King County yesterday acknowledged the organization has been hit hard financially by its decision to drop Planned Parenthood as a member agency in a dispute over abortions.

The controversy has resulted in a sharp decline in collections, the officials told 400 volunteers and representatives of member agencies at an emergency meeting in the Seattle Hilton Hotel.

As a result, they said, United ... today an all-out ... Way is ... media ... uses ... ments ... public ... full-p... Post- ... " ... inte... al ... cer... alw... Un...

Gilbert W. Anderson, volunteer chairman of the United Way board, said, "United Way was not told what to do by special interest ... of boycott."

services by contract, thus divorcing United Way from the abortion controversy.

Since 1977 it has been the policy of United Way of King County not to pay for abortions, ...

...troversy is hurting ...'s goal of collecting ...n, said Judy Runstad, ...ampaign chairwoman. ...now we've got some

...D WAY, Page A12

United Way sees slump in fund-raising effort after abortion dispute

by Joe Haberstroh
Times staff reporter

United Way plans a media blitz to try to stem a drop in this year's fund-raising efforts – a loss the organization attributes to the controversy over Planned Parenthood's recent decision to split with the agency.

Last year at this time, United Way had collected about $17.7 million, or 53 percent of its $33.4 million goal. So far this year, the agency has collected about $16 million, or 44 percent of its $36.7 million target for the campaign, which is to end Nov. 16.

Archbishop held a press conference demanding that Planned Parenthood resign from United Way or rescind its decision to do abortions. Right-wing religious groups tried to organize a campaign to eject PPSKC from United Way membership.

Nine months of negotiations between the affiliate and the United Way ensued. The affiliate negotiating team was made up of five executive committee members, the executive director, and legal counsel. At each meeting, at least three members of the team had to be present. Between negotiating sessions, reports, letters, and clippings were circulated to keep the entire team up to speed on ever-changing developments. The entire board was regularly apprised of the evolving situation.

Seeking Compromise. In order for the Seattle affiliate to remain a member of United Way (and continue to receive funds), United Way was demanding that Seattle set up two totally separate corporations—one for abortion services and one for the other program services—with separate facilities, staff, administration, and board members. Not surprisingly, this was exactly the way the Catholic Archdiocese wanted it. Seattle was willing to set up different corporations on paper, but with overlapping staff and board members, as dictated by the Planned Parenthood Federation guidelines.

Negotiations continued throughout the summer. At one point, four United Way officers asked to speak to the entire board because these funding fathers did not believe the negotiating committee was communicating the seriousness of United Way's intent. Board members spoke with one voice about their intent to serve clients effectively and efficiently—a goal which would have been impossible under the United Way plan.

OBSERVATION: Boards are composed of many people, yet to the public they have but one voice. The genius of the board of directors concept is that as a collection of many people it creates credibility. But for the board decisions to be understood by the community, they must stand for something and they must stand together.

United Way held its board meeting in September of 1988 to decide the status of the Seattle affiliate. At a press conference following the meeting, United Way announced that Seattle was being dropped from full membership, but United Way concocted a compromise alternative designed to appease the affiliate. Seattle would be offered a fee-for-service contract at the same funding level, as long as separate corporations were maintained. By this time, the press was following the story closely. The next day's headline in Seattle's daily paper read, "United Way Ousts Planned Parenthood."

D-Day at the Affiliate. The Seattle board met the following week to consider the offer. A fee-for-service contract turned out to be much different from a traditional "member" relationship in that it meant the affiliate would have to reapply each year for funds with no guarantee of receiving them. The board members faced a difficult decision. Could they afford to walk away from almost a half-million dollars and an 18-year relationship with United Way? Could they afford the hassle and expense of setting up two separate corporations with no guarantee of funds?

The current board chair and the immediate past chair (both of whom had been involved with the negotiations) set the agenda for the board meeting. The meeting began with a review of the history of negotiations. The executive director

---

Planned Parenthood in Seattle stood up and did the right thing. They lost over $400,000 but five years later PPSKC is raising close to $2.3 million.

outlined the pros and cons of each scenario. The staff business manager and vice president for operations addressed the programmatic and administrative impact of each plan.

Seattle's executive director, Lee Minto, remembers the meeting this way: "What a discussion ensued! Virtually everyone was there; virtually everyone spoke. Calm voices, reasoned voices, passionate voices, angry voices, and resolute voices. The board chair was determined that before she took a vote, everyone would understand the impact that rejecting the United Way offer would have on dramatically increasing the board's responsibility for fund raising . . . more discussion followed. At a critical juncture, a board member stood up and said, 'I think it is time for this board to take control of its own agenda again. For over a year we've let other people control what we spend our time and energy on. That needs to stop. Our patients need us, the community needs us. Let's get on with our work.' The motion to reject United Way's offer was passed with 36 positive and 2 negative votes, with an abstention from a brand new board member."

OBSERVATION: Leadership continuity and respect for history are crucial for good board decisions. Board membership turns over but good boards pass on institutional memory like a relay team hands off a baton. New board members are often asked to make hard decisions, even when much of the debate preceded their tenure on the board. Smooth transitions are assisted by comprehensive orientation sessions, good materials, and mentor relationships, matching old and new board members.

That afternoon, the chair of the Seattle board, chair-elect, past chair, and the executive director left the board meeting and walked into a room crammed with reporters from five television stations, eight radio stations, seven daily papers,

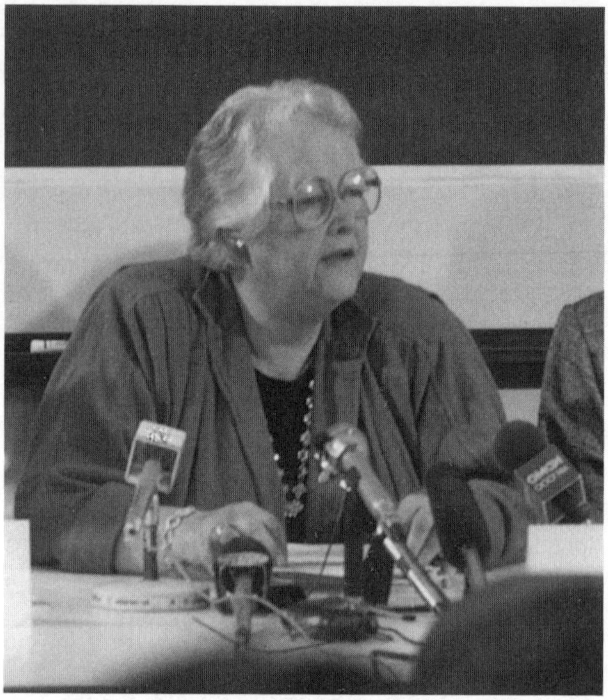

Lee Minto remembers the fall of 1988 as a watershed moment in the history of the Seattle affiliate.

the Associated Press, and United Press International. The board chair read a statement declaring, "We are deeply disappointed that United Way has set itself up to be perceived as United-only-if-you-agree-with-the-Catholic-Way." The chair went on to announce that the board of PPSKC would not accept the terms of a fee-for-service contract offered by United Way, thereby ending all relations between the two agencies.

The Reality Shock. With this decision, the board instantly gave itself a private fund-raising goal of over $800,000. In comments to the press, board members asked the community to support PPSKC and to continue their support of the United Way. Immediately the checks, calls, and letters began pouring in. The board's resource committee stepped up its activity, with board members coming in to help answer phones and handle the deluge of checks. The press helped by keeping the story alive both locally and nationally.

OBSERVATION: Planned Parenthood boards invariably underestimate the enormous reserve of support they have. When things are generally quiet, it becomes easy to hear just the noisy tactics of the shrill minority of the opposition. But when affiliates suffer a wrong in the pursuit of doing right, our supporters come out of the woodwork.

Between October and March, the Seattle affiliate's donors increased from 3,000 to over 14,000. More than 120 of the contributions were above the $1,000 mark, including one gift of $50,000. The fund-raising goal was exceeded in six months. The board instituted a policy of beginning fund raising for the budget year six months in advance to ensure a sold financial base for all programs.

OBSERVATION: Going through a crisis is a learning experience that teaches what new policies are needed. Boards celebrate victories, especially with close calls. Great boards learn and make changes so they'll never be as vulnerable again.

Because of its principled stand, PPSKC became the cause celebre in Seattle during the fall of 1988. More importantly, the affiliate's leaders learned that if they took a firm and unified commitment, obstacles that seemed insurmountable could be cleared and could take them to new heights. And four years later, the affiliate is thriving—and in 1992 is raising 2.3 million dollars a year.

CHAPTER EIGHT:

THE BOARD CHAIR:

Being at the Top Can Be Lonely or It Can Be the Best Seat in the House

"The chair's leadership job is to hold the lamp as high as possible so the board can see as far as possible; and then bring it down, so members can light their candle."

ANNE SAUNIER

A Tough Job. There *may* be a job more challenging than the chair or president of a Planned Parenthood board of directors, but it would be hard to find. There is never enough time, there are no easy recipes as to what to do, and the demands are never-ending. Why? Everyone seems to agree that the president's job is to lead the board, while the executive director leads the staff. Thus, if the board knows what it is supposed to do and does it, the president's job (i.e., leading the board) is manageable. If, on the other hand, the board is all over the place, dabbling here, interfering there . . . then being president is like being in charge of chaos.

For the board leader, the stakes are very high. Usually the president is a chief variable along with the executive director in creating excellence in the organization as a whole. Although we do not search for board leaders in the classified section of our local newspapers, if we did, the ad might look something like the example on page 85.

Amazingly enough, affiliate boards do find presidents who are often the best and the brightest in their communities. The explanation may be that although it is a tough job, it can be an exhilarating one. Being successful at it means that one is sustaining a well-run charity and also an agency capable of effecting social change. As board leader, an individual can make a discernible difference in a world in which impact is often hard to measure. The job can also prepare and tutor someone for other career opportunities.

> ***"[The Chair] . . . is a barrier-breaking visionary. An opportunity seeker and seizer. For his organization, he does not easily suffer a second-place position. He understands that a good loser—is a loser. There is an exhilaration in winning, but always for the common good. He admonishes his trustees to not be do-gooders, but doers of good."***
>
> **JEROLD PANAS**

> ***"The chairman ought to love the organization more than anyone else."***
>
> **KEN DAYTON**
> **Former Chairman and Chief Executive Officer of the Dayton Hudson Corporation**

A Basic Job Description. What can one reasonably expect the president to do? The following is a description of the president's "3 R's"—Requirements, Responsibilities, and Relationships. This is a condensed summary of a longer document that is found in *The Board Officer's Manual* published by the Planned Parenthood Western Region Assembly.

1. REQUIREMENTS
   - broad knowledge of the agency and personal commitment to the mission
   - demonstrated effectiveness as a leader within Planned Parenthood
   - adequate time to commit to leading the board, working with the executive director, and representing the affiliate nationally and regionally
   - ability to inspire board members to fulfill their roles as fund raisers, public affairs activists, planners, policy-makers, and fiscal stewards of the organization
   - ability to preside effectively at meetings of the board and to guide the board through its agenda

2. RESPONSIBILITIES
   - motivates and evaluates board functioning and is instrumental in planning for retreats and board education events
   - initiates and participates in the annual evaluation of the executive director

Wanted: Board President

A bright, articulate, high-energy leader with more than 10 years of experience in reproductive health care and advocacy. Must be able to take charge of a volunteer group already busy and often unavailable. Must effect change and direction without any real power by forging decisions from a diverse constituency who find it hard to agree on almost anything. Position is part time but applicant must be available all the time. Applicants must have two phone lines, an answering machine, a FAX machine, and a shredder. Computer skills preferred. Candidate should be able to leap tall buildings and walk on water. Compensation is competitive—no salary or benefits. Job lasts one to three years and will be terminated whether successful or not. Organization is an equal opportunity employer, and minorities are encouraged to apply.

Characteristics of Board Chairs:

The 1988 Survey.

The survey found that two-thirds of our Planned Parenthood board presidents at the time were female. 40 percent were 30 to 45 years old; 15 percent were 60 years or older; 38 percent did not have a job outside the home, 14 percent had a part-time job, and 47 percent had full-time jobs. Thus, almost two-thirds of the board had outside jobs which compete for time and attention with the responsibilities of being president of the affiliate board. And this is on top of the demands of families, ongoing commitments with other organizations, and the need for a little time for oneself.

Almost half (49 percent) of the board presidents had not been involved in Planned Parenthood before joining the affiliate board. Of those who had been seriously involved, 15 percent identified themselves as former volunteers and 20 percent had been on board committees, with fund-raising chair the most frequent apprentice role.

- monitors attendance at board meetings and initiates discussions with absent members
- ensures new member board orientation takes place and all members have requisite materials (e.g., strategic plans, policy manuals, recent minutes, board job descriptions, committee workplans)
- understands federation issues in a way to interpret the will of the board when representing affiliate with membership votes
- leads by example in fund raising and public affairs
- selects committee and task force chairs, and occasionally sits in on committee meetings in ex-officio capacity
- establishes with the executive director the agenda for board meetings

3. RELATIONSHIPS
- collaborative consultation and problem solving with the executive director, which should involve a high degree of candor, trust, and support
- create the same type of relationship with board officers, committee chairs, and members

Like all job descriptions, the expectations outlined above are somewhat idealized. No one could possibly be adept on each and every point. Board presidencies are positions that people grow into; they arrange the responsibilities to accentuate their strengths and minimize their weaknesses. What is essential is that the president have good "people skills," a respectful relationship with the executive director, the willingness to lead, and enough experience at Planned Parenthood to know the issues and the organization.

Leading Is Getting Harder. Most of the problems that an affiliate board president confronts are those that are generic to what some observers have called a "crisis in leadership." This crisis confronts all organizations—public and private, large and small. Leading an organization to change and to move forward is very hard, whether the venue is a Fortune 500 company, a division of government, or a Planned Parenthood affiliate. It is easy to fall into the trap of bureaucratic rules that blind the imagination, or the fear of failure that causes indecision and neutralizes progress, or the isolation from peer role models that leaves a leader dangling in the wind.

Simply stated, people often believe that leaders ought to know exactly where to go and that they need only to get their flock together, so the followers can get in line. But leadership doesn't work that way, nor does leadership of a board work that way. Board presidents lead by having their members set policy and plan strategically, in continuous interaction with the executive director's ideas and proposals. The board president orchestrates a group process that produces prudent decisions to guide the affiliate.

Brian O'Connell, an authority on leadership in the nonprofit sector, reminds us of the ancient Chinese proverb: "Those who lead well will know that their followers might say that they led themselves." Mahatma Gandhi similarly said, "There go my followers. I must get behind them for I am their leader." This is not to imply that the president should be an empty vessel with no idea of where to go or no clear cut sense of mission. Rather, as the leader-of-the-leaders, the president facilitates a board process that the members have bought into. The president doesn't have to know the right answers, but rather, the right questions, because in the final analysis, the best board leadership in our affiliates is provided by knowing how to frame the strategic questions and how to judge the answers that come from staff and board members.

"As chair, one of my biggest jobs was to give volunteers a kick in the pants and a shot in the arm."

ANNE SAUNIER

"It is essential that the leadership . . . help keep the dream out in front of people so that they see the relationship of such mundane things as budgets and annual plans and audits and evaluation in the context of the glorious outcomes that all of these people have come together to achieve . . . "

BRIAN O'CONNELL

Presidential Passion Is the Catalyst. Brian O'Connell is president of the Independent Sector, a national coalition of voluntary organizations, foundations, and corporations seeking to preserve and enhance American traditions of giving and volunteering. He is also the author of what has become a landmark book on nonprofit boards, *The Board Member's Book: Making a Difference in Voluntary Organizations.* In an interview, O'Connell offered critical insights about attributes of our best board leaders and the secrets of running a successful board. O'Connell describes the most important trait of a board president as: " . . . a deep sense of commitment—maybe even bordering on passion—for the cause, or at least some strong personal allegiance to the mission of this organization. I find those matters of personal commitment to be more important and fundamental than other aspects."*

It is evident from O'Connell's experience that the chief assets of a board president are enthusiasm and passion for the dream. The president's enthusiasm will be contagious to everyone on the board and leadership staff. The combination of passion along with the ability to lead debates that culminate in action is what defines first rate leadership. The board president might be titled "Resident Dream Manager." When the *direction of the dream* best serves the organization's real owners—patients, donors, and communities—then the board has done its job. Once the board has accomplished this, staff members can add their unique contributions to organizational success by creating productivity measures and business plans and by giving attention to details.

Board Meeting Times:

The 1988 Survey.

The survey results indicate that a majority of the boards meet on Tuesday, Wednesday, and Thursday, only three percent meet on the weekend, and none meet on Friday. 35 percent meet at the lunch hour, 26 percent meet late afternoon, 29 percent in the evening, and one early-bird board meets at 9:00 a.m. Although it was not a survey question, board meeting times have been altered as affiliates either merge or expand to become more geographically scattered. This trend tends to doom the Wednesday-at-noon tradition, common when affiliates were more often a single, local community agency. If this regionalization continues, it will most certainly create an era in which boards will end up meeting on the weekend or for more extended periods in the evening.

> ***[To be the president] "means encouraging people to feel comfortable with discussion and debate with each other. The person in the chair in other contexts may be a tiger or individual performer, a slasher, a doer, but the role requires emphasizing group process . . . "***
>
> **BRIAN O'CONNELL**

Styles of Board Leadership. Although individual personality traits naturally play a role, many board leaders have definite styles owing in large part to the particular environment of Planned Parenthood. In affiliate boards, one often finds a highly developed appreciation for democracy and an emphasis on the need for effective group process. Board members often don't want to offend their peers, and board presidents seem to want to hear from everybody (twice). The organizational culture of Planned Parenthood does not tend to produce macho, charismatic autocrats who command by giving orders and asking followers to fetch. Rather, the successful board chair quietly keeps attention on things most important, forges decisions from thoughtful debate, and enables progress without having to manipulate the board to accept his or her predetermined course of action.

> ***"Autocrats kill vitality."***
>
> **NORAH HOLMGREN**

* Reprinted with permission from *The Board Member's Book: Making a Difference in Voluntary Organizations,* copyright © 1985 by Brian O'Connell, The Foundation Center, 79 Fifth Ave., New York, NY 10003-3050.

The Moment of Truth: the Board Meeting. The task that many board presidents dread—one often overlooked in articles and even in board manuals—is the board meeting itself. Many of the techniques of running good board meetings are the same as running any meeting—solid preparation, a clear agenda, a method of recording action taken, etc. But board meetings can't just replicate a business meeting of the senior staff of a local corporation. Board meetings have something in common with legislative debate. Members see themselves as representing values and constituencies. Thus, they do not speak just as individuals expressing their own views about a certain issue. They have the more complicated task of trying to get in touch with what clients would want or which course of action best serves a value (e.g., privacy, choice, self-determination, etc.) they determine as most critical. The two governance mainstays of creating strategy and policy are not always obvious, and they often don't emerge swiftly during meetings. Thus, board presidents use a much broader array of skills than if they were just gray suits with power ties and jeweled Rolexes.

The other confounding dynamic is that the board exists as something you can see and hear for a limited time only, from the sound of the gavel calling the meeting to order to the stroke that marks adjournment. Whereas an executive director can bring management staff back the next day if they cannot finish work on time or if they do not get it done right, the board president almost never has that luxury. Within the tight confines of the meeting, the board president must make good work happen. "The chair's job is not to problem solve," as Anne Saunier has said, "but to know the mechanism to get the board to do it." She must simultaneously be maestro, taskmaster, facilitator, diplomat, and task fanatic. The suggestions in figure ten on page 90 should help board presidents make their meetings effective, interesting, and productive.

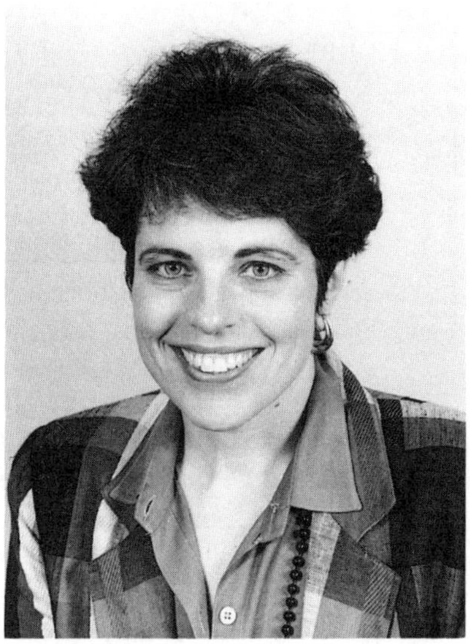

"One of the worst moments of board planning is when the board spends all its time and energy trying to smooth the feathers of a member who doesn't like to plan. The result is that everyone walks away unenthused."

ROSANN WISMAN
Executive Director
Planned Parenthood of Metropolitan Washington, D.C.

"The biggest difference between being a board member and being president . . . as a member, I often waited to get fed; but as the president, I had to do the feeding."

CATHY FRANK

Making Board Meetings Work. Since there are few second chances, it is vital to get things done right the first time. Before a board meeting, most presidents have an agenda-planning session with their

FIGURE TEN:

Four "Metal" Groups that Make for Better Board Meetings

1. **Golden Rule:** *Keep meetings as informal as possible to encourage open, honest discussions.* At the same time, board leaders should also possess a good working knowledge of Robert's Rules of Order and basic parliamentary procedures, particularly when guiding tricky board discussions. However, straight talk, devoid of complex parliamentary maneuvers, usually makes for better decisions than those that have escaped the torture of three "points of order," two "tablings," and one "friendly," but "non-germane" amendment.

2. **Silver Lining:** *Do not require unanimous decisions.* If the board always strives for consensus, it means that precious time will be spent trying to convince the dissenters to go along with the majority, often robbing other issues of their due attention. Good boards can manage split votes and get on to the next task. This is not to say that one should blithely ignore the thoughts of the out-voted minority. Give them the forum to express their view and don't browbeat them to conform with the majority.

3. **Brass Ring:** *Run board meetings with common sense and good group process skills.* Members need to be courteous and respectful to each other. From time to time, it may be useful to use skill-building exercises to teach the art of assertively speaking up in the group, while at the same time respecting other people's points of view.

4. **Iron Glove:** *Avoid factions and personal politics.* Good boards are composed of persons who do not vote as factions (e.g., not as education committee members, everyone from a certain county) and who do not defer unduly to other members of the board just because they are wealthy, wield power in the local community, have been around a long time, or have put in the most hours with the affiliate.

executive. Here they jointly decide what time-driven tasks must be done (such as authorizations and corporate approvals), what things are most important to do, and what other things would be nice to do if enough time remains. The president must have sufficient command of the issues to be discussed so he/she can keep the board focused and moving forward, especially as side-tracks inevitably emerge. In turn, the executive must anticipate the organization's needs and use this preboard meeting as an opportunity to brief the president thoroughly.

Preparation for a board meeting is helped if there is a yearly schedule that lays out those overall goals and objectives that the board must accomplish at a certain time (e.g., the budget, board self-assessment). For example, if one is aware that the next board meeting will include a thorough review of the annual financial audit, one can skip the treasurer's report if time is tight. For many boards, repetition wastes time and creates frustration. (Incidentally, in some organizations this agenda-planning task is occasionally performed by the entire executive committee. That strikes me as an inappropriate diffusion of leadership that may also tempt a handful of board members to get too far ahead of the board as a whole.)

"There are ways to keep the trustee's battery at a state of constant positive charge. One is to make certain that the agenda at each meeting provides for stimulating discussion and an opportunity for a major decision. Trustees must feel a sense of worth and importance to the organization."

JEROLD PANAS

Time Management. The tendency in Planned Parenthoods to encourage democratic participation in discussions is valuable. But if the president allows discussion to drag out, it will be difficult to extract crisp, definitive decisions. Most presidents find it useful to assign exact time limits for each specific agenda item so there will be adequate opportunity to act on all items requiring discussion. While chair cannot always exactly adhere to the time goals, this process does allow him/her to anticipate time problems and avoid having the most critical issues tabled to a later date simply because all the earlier items took longer than expected. In addition, some effective presidents have a cardinal rule that, except in the most extraordinary circumstances, the meeting must begin and end as advertised (plus or minus no more than 15 minutes). This procedure disciplines board discussion and helps guard against one of the biggest sins of board work: voting something up or down in haste simply because the hour is late and fatigue has set in.

"The board room should be comfortable, facilitate work, be free of distractions. I've seen an affiliate really make it work, with key charts posted to the wall as reminders of the bottom line."

BOB BLOMBERG
Regional Director
Western Regional Office PPFA

Room Aesthetics and Physical Layout. The president must take charge of running the meeting. Many presidents find it useful to have their table or podium set apart from other board members so that focus and sight lines are concentrated on the president. Usually, some modified oval seating arrangement works best. Comfort is important. Chairs (the seat, not the presiding officer) should be supportive and writing surface available. A room with windows to the outside world is preferable. This meeting room is the board's worksite; ergonomics matter. If you need proof, just think back to the last meeting you attended where you couldn't see who was talking or you sat in those one-size-fits-all school desk/chairs.

Often a president will position the executive next to himself, thereby clustering the leadership. It is also best to have presenters come to the front when they speak. If the board is large, it is helpful for the president to stand up occasionally so his position is clear and he

"Members who don't speak out are the biggest problem. Allow for disagreement. The worst thing is chronic abstaining."

ETHELYN BISHOP

can see the group as a whole, more easily acknowledging people when they seek their turn to speak.

Varying the Format and Subject Areas. The best meetings are the ones that offer a change of pace. They may incorporate different subject themes, varied group process styles, and many different presenters. Good meetings should have something for the head and something for the heart. For example, a report on suggested bylaw changes could be followed by a staff counselor's briefing about how the issue of incest is handled when it comes up in a patient interview.

The *subjects* at hand should ideally be addressed in a variety of ways, so that the meeting is a blend of presentations, discussions, and debate. For example, a board meeting might include:

- DISCUSSION of pragmatic business issues (e.g., Should we change investment brokers because of last year's disappointing yields?);
- DEBATE about an aspect of Planned Parenthood's mission and future (e.g., Is there any reason to believe we'd be better off if we merged with our neighboring affiliate?);
- PRESENTATION by staff, followed by board discussion, on an ethical quandary that needs board policy (e.g., What are the advantages and disadvantages of noting positive AIDS test results in a patient's chart?).

The *group process* should include both reports (from committees, work groups, outside experts) and open-ended debate. Many boards find it beneficial occasionally to break down into smaller groups, divide an issue into component parts, and encourage participation by less vocal members. The board meeting also is more effective when discussions and presentations are not dominated by the same members meeting after meeting. The advantages are that different personalities make the meeting more interesting, the chair gets a chance to rest and gather his/her thoughts, and the group gets evidence that leadership is shared, not the exclusive domain of a small clique.

Focusing Staff Roles. Because this is the board's meeting, staff should not carry or dominate the agenda. Of course, there are always key facts that must be provided by the executive and management staff, since the board needs full disclosure of pertinent points to make effective policy decisions. But staff should prepare the president and committee chairs ahead of time so that staff input can be kept to a minimum during the actual meeting. If a board needs the staff to explain the issues being discussed, this may be a clue that the board is getting too involved in the details of affiliate operations.

> ***"Boards must not fall into the dilemma or busy trap of not having the opportunity to discuss and debate key issues with staff management. It is in these exchanges where the really good ideas are created."***
>
> **DR. KENNETH EDELIN**

While staff should not dominate board meetings, it is critical for all senior level managers to attend the meeting so that the board work does not take on an air of secrecy. In addition, management staff must experience firsthand the tone and texture of the board's deliberation, which helps them considerably when they put these policies into practice. Several Planned Parenthood boards also have found it useful to have a staff member draft the minutes of the meeting so that the secretary of the board can more fully participate in deliberations.

Efficiency Techniques. Board chairs learn immediately that there is never enough meeting time to handle everything comprehensively. Several techniques are commonly used to expedite board meetings. *Consent agendas* are written explanations of certain routine matters given to board members in advance, with no further discussion, unless a member asks to have the item moved to the regular agenda. *Monitoring reports* on key operational areas – fund raising, service data, financial statements – are written in a way that emphasizes outcome and not process. For example, if fund raising is ahead of goal, it is not essential for the board to know why the spring event was changed from a book auction to a charity ball. These reports should be discussed only if a serious problem exists that the board needs to correct. *Executive summary capsules* placed prominently at the top of committee minutes serve to highlight actions taken and key points for consideration. Such a summary helps to focus attention on the essentials.

> ***"If you don't want board members involved in the daily business of the organization, why give them an invitation by reporting to them about daily activities?"***
>
> **ANONYMOUS ADMINISTRATOR**

Mid-course Corrections. If the board meets in large time blocks, it is a good idea to break mid-meeting. This gives everyone a chance to stretch, get some air, clear their minds, and simply socialize. It also gives the chair an opportunity to consult privately with the executive or with upcoming presenters. For example, if an agenda item is being blocked or is floundering, a time-out allows the president to determine if the item should be held over to a future meeting or if it can be resolved by a private consultation with the key players. This break time also gives the president an opportunity to do a time check and to inform members that they are going to have more (or, usually, less) time than originally planned. It also allows for small group discussion on what has happened in the meeting and its effects. One-on-one conversations may permit certain board members to get their questions answered without a full board discussion.

> ***"The relationship between the Board President and the Executive Director is one of responsible partnership. Like all human partnerships, this one has moments of tension and difficulty. Mutual trust, respect and courtesy will go a long way toward minimizing any difficulties that arise."***
>
> *Board Papers* **PPFA, Western Region**

> ***"To make the role of the board president really meaningful, the incoming president should have a clear notion of the single-most important thing that they want to accomplish in their term of office. And if they achieve this goal, there is nothing that feels quite so rewarding."***
>
> **DR. KENNETH EDELIN**

Post-meeting Debriefing. The president and executive director should meet after the board meeting to figure out exactly what happened, how to communicate the decisions that were made, and what additional information is needed before the next meeting for items that were not resolved. This get-together should happen as soon as possible, because a hectic, fast-paced board meeting is very complicated to reconstruct after much time has elapsed. Both parties also may use this time to critique constructively the results of the meeting and to provide performance feedback to each other. Critiquing the president is often awkward for the executive, but because chairing the board meeting is so important, the president needs immediate and specific feedback. This process is probably best understood as a mutual peer review, where good performance is appraised and applauded, while poor performance is critiqued by the leadership partner. Executive directors and presidents are in the best position to critique and coach each other. There is usually no better way to improve.

Preparing New Board Presidents. Nonprofit boards are just about the only organizational entities that turn over their leader, president, or chair after two years, often just when the person is getting good at the job. This practice is rationalized as a way to bring a new and refreshing perspective. Unfortunately, this revolving door leadership can reduce a great board to a mediocre board because board leadership seems to be in perpetual transition. In addition, boards always have a freshman or sophomore at the helm. Some boards have found creative ways to cope with this revolving door leadership.

- Have a formal president-elect system so the next president can be apprenticing for a year before taking on the job. Also, keep the most recent past-president on the board, so he/she is accessible to consult with the new president.
- Do not select an unproven or unknown person for the presidency.
- Find someone who has served on the board and knows the organization well. Also, do not be tempted to pick a person as president just because he/she has worked hard and it seems to be his/her turn. Suitability for the presidency must be based on demonstrated performance and leadership potential.
- Give presidents instant access to attend regional and national meetings. Encourage them to go to the Planned Parenthood Leadership Institutes New Board Presidents' Workshop. Provide adequate board travel funds. If you cannot afford this, you need to reassess your affiliate's financial priorities.
- Encourage former board presidents to stay involved so they can mentor new presidents. In one affiliate, this informal group refers to itself as the Beached Whale Club and gets together occasionally with the current president to swap stories, seek advice, and share perspectives.

Time Commitment:

The 1988 Survey.

Board presidents were asked about the average amount of time they spend in their Planned Parenthood role. Ten hours a week was the average: eight hours in the role of president and two hours on other Planned Parenthood matters, like fund raising and advocacy. Within the 10 hours, presidents attend an average of one committee meeting a week. The presidents also reported that they talked with their executive for an average of just over one hour each week.

"The board president must be elected on competency—not as a reward for surviving."

NORAH HOLMGREN

In Summary. The board president has a demanding job with only about one long working day a week to get it done. Time management becomes essential. Furthermore, the president's leadership role is challenging. One need only look back at Chapter Two to see what experts feel are the challenges and difficulties in trying to get a board to succeed. But as board expert Arthur Frantzreb has written, "[Presidents] . . . must dream of what the board and organization may become in spite of evidence to the contrary." The ability to keep the Planned Parenthood dream alive testifies to the genius of the voluntary organization, with its volunteer leader at the top.

"Two wrong reasons to be a board president; a friend pressures them or board is so desperate, they are thrown into a job they aren't ready for."

ETHELYN BISHOP

CHAPTER NINE:

THE PARTNERSHIP:

Board President and Executive Director

"The president is not the executive director's superior—that's the entire board's role. I think working partner is the way to view the relationship."

ANNE SAUNIER

"The best and most dynamic affiliates have aggressive staff that push and boards that, as part of the larger community, act as a brake."

ANNE SAUNIER

Organizational Health Starts at the Top. In evaluating an organization's health, one of the first questions to ask is, "How are board and staff relations?" If the answer is "great," manifestations of the agency's good health will abound in every facet of organizational life; if the answer is "terrible," multiple symptoms probably will prevail and sickness will spread throughout the affiliate's various functions. The climate for board/staff relationships starts right at the top, with the working relationship between the board president and the executive director.

"The C.E.O. and the board president act as a bridge for maintaining good working relationships . . . but . . . people who try to build bridges must be prepared to be walked on."

VAUGHN KELLER

Respect and trust for each other along with a compatible partnership between the two heads of the agency are prerequisites of affiliate success. This partnership does not just happen automatically. It requires diligence and open communication. The objective is that both parties can act as each other's first-line support system. If these two people cannot be there for each other, then trouble can brew.

"A good board president needs to see the president's role in leadership as leading and motivating the board, setting the charges for committee chairs and investing heavily in the planning and monitoring process. It is a great temptation for board presidents to become too involved in personnel matters and internal stuff, an understandable problem since the president works so intimately with the executive director . . . "

LYN REYNOLDS
Former Executive Director
Planned Parenthood
of Santa Clara County

These two jobs of board president and executive director are at the very top of the hierarchy of the voluntary and paid staff sectors of the affiliates. They are "lightning rod" jobs that, Vaughn Keller suggests, will inevitably generate criticism and be the target of some pot shots from the organization's multiple constituencies—even if (and perhaps *especially* if) they are good leaders. This happens because leadership requires making some unpopular decisions, taking risks, and making changes. In the long haul, these leadership decisions often prove to be prophetic and terrific; in the short term, they almost never cause the people in charge to win popularity polls. This happens because the driving force behind leadership is to do the right thing, not necessarily the thing that makes people feel good. But as Harry S Truman said, "If you can't stand the heat, get out of the kitchen." Because these jobs are very difficult, it is imperative that both these partners be there to support and protect each other.

In addition to seeking help from each other, the board president and the executive director can look to other support systems. The ex-

The Partners Speak:

The 1988 Survey.

There was much agreement among the board presidents when they were asked to differentiate between their leadership and that of the executives. Presidents and executive directors repeatedly responded that the biggest distinction was between *whom* they lead: The president leads the board, the executive leads the staff. Some survey answers were particularly notable: At the board meetings themselves, "the president is more motivational, the executive director more informational," whereas at most other times the situation was reversed. Several presidents talked about their relationships with their board members. For instance, " . . . many feel more able to confide in me than the executive director." Another president suggested why this occurs, "I am one of the board (a volunteer) and they identify with me."

ecutive director can turn to buddy and mentor systems for new executive directors within the federation, the National Executive Director Council of Planned Parenthood, and other local nonprofit executives. Although fewer support systems exist for volunteer leaders, they have begun to emerge. Board presidents in Planned Parenthood have formed the Affiliate Presidents Council. Additionally, many presidents cherish and cultivate the informal connections they make at board presidents' training workshops, annual Federation meetings, and regional spring conferences. However, there is no substitute for the primary support relationship of the executive and president. It must be clear, cordial, and trusting. And when it is not, it needs to be fixed ASAP.

"Nonprofits waste uncounted hours debating who is superior and who is subordinate—board or executive officer. The answer is that they must be colleagues. Each has a different part to play. Their tasks are complementary. Thus, each has to ask, What do I owe the other, not—as board and executive officers tend to do—What does the other one owe me? The two have to work as one team of equals."

PETER DRUCKER

The Power Debate: Who Really Is in Charge? Although the dynamics of personality and individual styles of the executive director and board president occasionally cause stress, a more fundamental tension underlies the relationship—one that sometimes grows and causes board-staff conflicts in all types of nonprofit organizations.

> ***"It is not necessary for executive directors and boards to walk in lockstep or to consistently view the world from the same perspective. On the other hand, an institution works best when executive directors and board presidents have a common understanding of job priorities and the stresses created by meeting those priorities, not when its leadership is at loggerheads."***
>
> **—excerpt from *An Analysis of Planned Parenthood Executive Director Turnover in 1990.***

The dilemma can be simply stated. People within nonprofit organizations and people on the outside looking in have a very fundamental need to know who is in charge and who is the ultimate decision-maker. Is it the board or is it the executive director? In nonprofits, much of the discussion of this fundamental question is confusing double-speak. We tend to give answers that explicitly say "both" or implicitly suggest "neither." Nonprofits too often display a classic table of organization that looks like this:

FIGURE ELEVEN:

The Theoretical Table of Organization

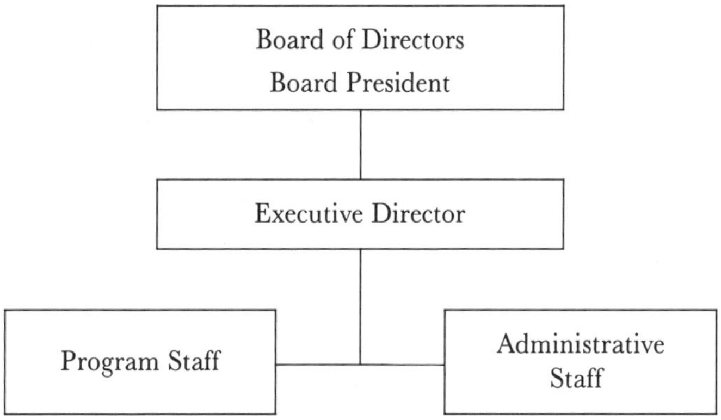

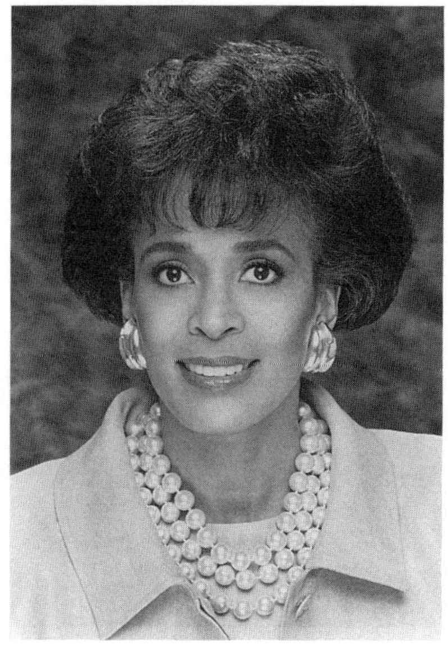

"The power of information that the C.E.O. holds is enormous . . . executive directors must handle this power responsibly."

FAYE WATTLETON

In this structure, the board president is prominently placed as the highest ranking corporate officer and thus the person who is ultimately in charge. This configuration aptly captures the legal aspect of the board with the authority to hire and fire the executive director. But relegating the executive director – the person who is seen by 95 percent of the world as the leader of the organization – to the secondary layer invites confusion. It can disempower an executive director, turning her into a passive participant "waiting for the board to tell me what to do next." Neither Lee Iacocca nor the Pope runs his shop in this manner. Furthermore, this configuration misrepresents the organization's actual behavior and the process of how things work. If one observed the way power and authority are actually practiced in many nonprofits, the relationship might look like this:

FIGURE TWELVE:

The Table of Organization in Actual Practice

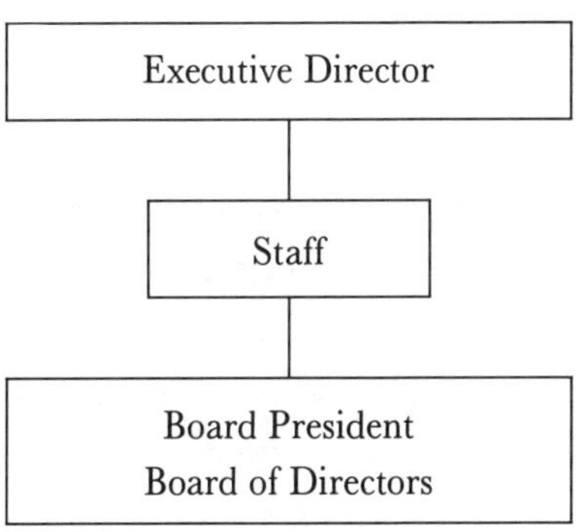

In this structure, the executive director calls the shots, staff makes things happen, and the board members are warm bodies assigned primarily to observer status. The sad reality is that many boards, and thus their leaders, do not understand their power and are accurately pictured at the bottom of the heap. Boards that are adrift, that never seem to know exactly what they are supposed to do, limit themselves to secondary (and quite often, peripheral) tasks. While theoretically retaining the ultimate power of firing and hiring the executive, they usually are in no position to exercise even this responsibility until the affiliate is in a full-blown crisis.

Distinct But Shared Power. Neither of the models pictured in figures eleven and twelve is particularly helpful. My contention is that the best way to visualize the ideal power and structural relationship would be to flip the table of organization on its side. Thus, it would look like this:

FIGURE THIRTEEN:

Shared Power Model

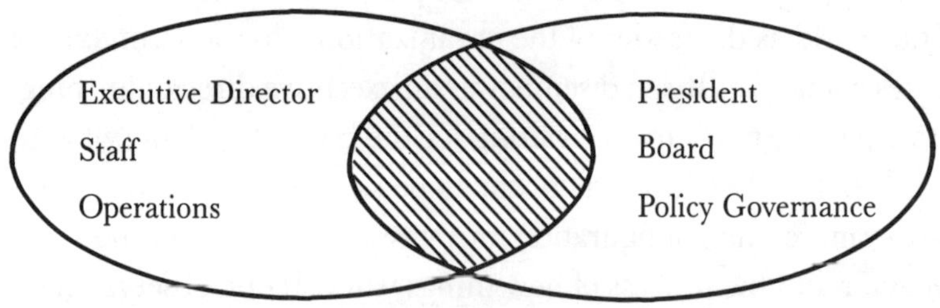

This is a shared power model that is collegial and parallel. It diffuses the need to assert a traditional superior-subordinate relation of board and staff. Each leader has a clear, discrete domain where she is in charge *and* a shared domain where, together, they lead the organization by mutual consent. The executive director leads the staff; the president leads the board. The executive director *manages* by planning, organizing, and evaluating all aspects of affiliate operations; the president and board *govern* by setting policy and long-term strategies. In some nonprofits, this type of relationship is reflected in changes in the titles used to refer to the top staff and volunteer positions. The executive director is now being called "president" of the corporation, while the top board officer is called the "chairperson" of the board. Although this terminology is not absolutely essential, it does better capture the essence of the jobs and parallels that of private sector counterparts.

"The ability of board and staff to operate in a 'we' mode versus a 'they' mode exists in all our very best affiliates."

GERALD COOK
Regional Director
Southern Region, PPFA

In this model, there is also an important interface in which both sides share power. The executive director recommends policies and advances strategic planning ideas for board consideration; conversely, the board creates a system of monitoring operations, evaluating the implementation of policies, analyzing current results against planning benchmarks, and appraising the performance of the chief executive officer. Margaret Kantner, a trainer of volunteers for the United Way, has written about how boards and executive directors must understand their roles to avoid problems. She contends that although there are some clear cut lines of exclusive domain, more often "... [most issues] will have both idea and action components and will require the board and the executive to collaborate in the decision-making. *The board makes the value judgments; management takes action."*

"Realistically, the executive director will be comfortable with a decision and ready to move ahead before the board will be ready to do the same."

FAYE WATTLETON

"Probably the trait most valued by executive directors, though, is one of trust and confidence. An anxious president usually means an uninformed one, and usually the anxieties stem from a lack of experience with management and fiscal policies and procedures. And, of course, the president and the executive director are partners, sharing responsibility and each managing his own piece of the action, so they have to meet often, keep no secrets, share what they know and like the job."

LYN REYNOLDS

The region of shared power is that in which policy and strategic planning are translated into business and operations. Both leaders negotiate to ensure that sufficient progress is occurring on both fronts, at an agreed upon pace, so that neither side is getting too far in front of the other. Both leaders should also make sure that fund raising and advocacy are running smoothly. As described in Chapter Seven, these two functions have both board and staff actively involved out in the community, so it is critical to communicate and coordinate so that overlap is minimized. If left unmanaged, the shared work (with its potential advantages) disintegrates into a muddy area of ambiguous roles and activities.

Of course, the organization will always have its formal sphere in

"When I visit affiliates that are risk takers and successful, I always find a board and a chief executive officer where there is mutual trust and respect."

DR. KENNETH EDELIN

which the board sits on top and its informal sphere in which staff dominates with their power of expertise and superior access to information. What I am suggesting, however, is to avoid skirmishes over where the absolute power lies, which is a win-lose proposition (i.e., for the executive director to assert her superior position, the board must adopt the subordinate role . . . and vice versa). The secret is to understand that *each* leader has a discrete domain of ultimate responsibility. For the president, it is the board of directors and the functions of strategic planning and policy development; for the executive director, it is the staff and the operations of administration and program. But it is the sphere of shared responsibility (see Figure Thirteen), in which strategy and operations are shared by mutual consent, that exemplifies this leadership partnership in action.

The Need for Ground Rules. If, as Frost says, "Good fences make good neighbors," then good ground rules make for good leadership partners. Every affiliate needs to have defined ground rules to assist an effective president-executive relationship. Although many of these guidelines may intuitively emerge, it is better if they are understood, agreed upon, and written down as part of the affiliate's board policies. This allows them to be applied consistently and repeated every time one of the partners changes. Often affiliates can go for years without needing to resort to rules, but if a serious problem emerges, it is a godsend to have them established.

In the partner relationship of the executive director and board president, each party needs to be able to expect certain behaviors from the other so that each can do his or her own job. These are as follows:

FIGURE FOURTEEN:

Ground Rules for the Leadership Duo

MUTUAL EXPECTATIONS

1. No surprises
2. Hard work
3. Public solidarity / private critique
4. No need to blame

WHAT EXECUTIVE DIRECTOR NEEDS FROM PRESIDENT

5. Wisdom more than information
6. Management of the board
7. Personal and professional respect
8. Unwavering support from a coach

WHAT PRESIDENT NEEDS FROM EXECUTIVE DIRECTOR

9. Steady quest for excellence
10. Unadorned information
11. Empowerment of the board

With these ground rules set and followed, the organizational leaders have a covenant with each other. Like all interdependent relationships, this one demands that both parties work hard to make good on their vows to each other. While it is true that they are not "marrying each other 'til death do them part," they are definitely living together (so to speak) for a couple of years.

> ***"The president's job is very time-consuming, but don't fight it . . . organize it. Grab every opportunity, for it is more than a fair exchange."***
>
> **CATHY FRANK**

Mutual Expectations. There are certain behaviors that both parties must reasonably expect from each other:

- NO SURPRISES. The board leader must always be honest and must bring to the executive's attention things the executive needs to know, especially real or perceived mistakes made by the executive director. Whenever a significant issue has arisen (such as major board dissatisfaction with the executive director or inappropriate staff interaction with the board) the executive director needs to know virtually the minute after the president knows. The board president in turn expects "no surprises" from the executive director. Nothing is likely to cause more trouble than a president hearing about a major trouble area in the affiliate from anyone other than the executive director.

- HARD WORK. The board president's role cannot and should not be full time. But in urgent situations, she must make herself available from morning to night. A lazy or overcommitted president robs the board. The same holds true for the executive director. A low energy, out-the-door-by-four executive director models what will become part of the organization's culture—namely, staff doesn't need to work very hard around here. Lax standards for work rob the nonprofit of its major competitive advantage over private industry or government service: namely, employees willing to push hard and pull long hours because of belief in the overall cause.

- PUBLIC SOLIDARITY / PRIVATE CRITIQUE. In order for two-part leadership to work, it is imperative that the board president and executive director speak with one voice in public. At the very least, they should not pointedly contradict each other. They do not have to agree on everything, but they must respect each other and use every opportunity to support each other's work. In *private* meetings, they can and should critique each other and hash out major differences of opinion concerning the affiliate. Problems, differences of opinion, and differing priorities should not be allowed to fester but should be brought up and discussed.

"A college president told me the other day that the board chairperson who can smile when things go wrong . . . has thought of a dean to blame it on!"

JEROLD PANAS

- NO NEED TO BLAME. To make this relationship work, both parties must not automatically blame each other's constituency for affiliate deficiencies. The executive must be particularly sensitive in this area. Some executives castigate the board for the affiliate's inability to fund raise or plan strategically, cavalierly covering up serious doubts about their own skills with the excuse, "The board won't do it." Occasionally this may be true. But it is far more likely that the executive is masking his/her worries about adequately providing the board with the tools and staff support to be successful fund raisers or planners. Finger-pointing is the worst way to identify problems and generate solutions.

What Executive Directors Need from Presidents. The board as a collective whole is the boss of the executive director, but the president is the singular individual who manifests the board's desires and duties. She needs to be the messenger that keeps seeing "the big picture"; she needs to referee disputes and inspire her members; she is the person who interacts most with the executive director. The C.E.O. needs the following fundamental points from the board president:

- WISDOM MORE THAN INFORMATION. Executives are overloaded with information and swamped with data. Most of the time, they do not need more. They do need the president to help sort out the less important from the essential, the big issues from the minutiae; and they need advice on how to engage the board in moving the affiliate forward.

- MANAGEMENT OF THE BOARD. Board management is the unique role of the president. The executive director needs the president to correct inappropriate board behavior and to reward excellence. If the executive director tries to step in, he/she is entering a mine field. Not only does the executive director work for the board (and not the other way around), but the executive director who "manages" the board is overstepping the lines of authority of the formal organization. Ideally a board will manage itself, but the chair must not be afraid to troubleshoot problems and referee disputes. In some instances boards have gone from good to bad at lightning speed and often the culprit has been a president unwilling or unavailable to nip emerging problems in the bud.

"Any institution . . . which has an all-powerful chairman or a weak C.E.O. is an institution in trouble."

KEN DAYTON

- PERSONAL AND PROFESSIONAL RESPECT. Executive directors need their presidents to set a tone of trust and respect for the competence and credibility of staff. The board must not see itself principally as overseer of the help. In some nonprofits, there is a thinly veiled attitude that staff members will not do what they are supposed to do unless they are ridden hard and watched constantly. The board president must rid the organization of this military mentality and keep offending board members out of staff members' hair.

"As trustees, we are there . . . to support, encourage, challenge, stimulate and help that professional who we pick to lead our endeavor. If every board could see its role as that . . . we would have far more dynamic institutions, far stronger professional executives . . ."

KENNETH DAYTON
at the Independent Sectors
1987 Professional Forum

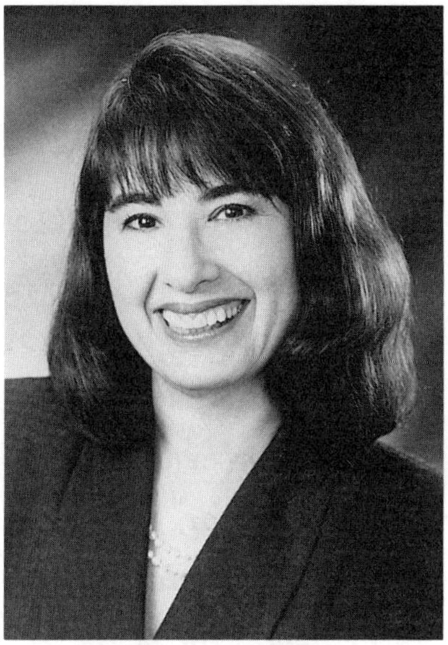

"Boards are very delicate ecosystems: one bad actor can make things miserable."

GLORIA FELDT
Executive Director
Planned Parenthood of
Central and Northern Arizona

- UNWAVERING SUPPORT OF AN EMPATHETIC ADVOCATE. The executive director needs the board president to provide compliments when deserved, corrective coaching when necessary, advocacy for generous compensation, and sufficient autonomy to run the ship. Additionally, more than one superlative president has run interference for, or deflected criticism from, an executive director under pressure. The president must make sure that the terms and conditions of employment are enabling and provide incentives for the executive director. This is what the author and management expert, Ken Blanchard, would call "catching the executive doing something good." John Carver calls it "giving the executive the space to run the organization" and even "providing the freedom to fail."

What Presidents Need from Executive Directors. It is virtually impossible for a president to do a good job if the affiliate has a mediocre or weak executive. Conversely, if the executive director delivers the goods in the next three areas, the president can be a star.

- ORGANIZATIONAL EXCELLENCE. A president needs an executive director who is willing to be held accountable and to lead the organization. The executive director sets the tone within the affiliate. If he settles for "ordinary" results and outcomes, that is

"A good executive director should never bring a proposal in completely cold; get a sense of the concerns and try to address them. Talk early on to a board member who may be opposed, or, at least, is good at playing the devil's advocate."

ROSANN WISMAN

what he'll get; if he expects and personally strives for excellence, outstanding results often ensue. He must lead by example, taking the toughest lobbying assignment or fund-raising call and demanding the best from everyone connected to the affiliate. This provides the organization with a high benchmark for which to strive. Walking the walk and talking the talk of leadership is the executive director's most important contribution.

"Excellence is your organization's lifeline. It is the only answer to apathy and inertia. Once it becomes the expected standard of performance, it develops a life of its own, a fiercely driving and motivating philosophy of operation. It guides everything you do. Excellence is a state of mind put into action. When a climate of excellence exists in your organization, all things are success-driven. Your staff work, volunteer leadership, finances, and program — they all feel the impact and the stimulation and the inspiration."

JEROLD PANAS

- UNADORNED INFORMATION. Board presidents and board members need basic, unadorned and pertinent data so that their actions are sufficient to the needs of any situation. The executive director can easily manipulate the board process if he withholds basic information or puts an overly gloomy or overly cheery spin on his reports. This imperative to disclose fully is especially important when it is the hardest to do, with bad or threatening news. Many outside observers have blamed boards for failing to react quickly when an affiliate starts having serious problems, but more often than not, their executive never adequately described the seriousness of the situation. In some ways, this is only natural. The executive may be understandably embarrassed or guilty about things that are going badly and may fear that if all is known, he will lose his job. But executives must do everything possible to resist the temptation to withhold information. Good boards do not look for scapegoats; they appreciate getting the facts of the situation.

They need to know everything there is to know soon enough to avoid a crisis.

- EMPOWERMENT OF THE BOARD. The board president needs an executive director who wants the board to govern, to challenge his assumptions, and to be a "player" in the shared leadership of the affiliate. The executive must truly *want* a powerful and wise board, if he is going to get one. There are a thousand ways for the executive to create a weak, rubber-stamping board. He simply can never send up really important or substantial proposals. He can guard information so closely that boards have no alternative but to either acquiesce or rebel. He can establish himself as the all-knowing professional (hiding behind layer upon layer of technical jargon) and can dismiss questions or challenges simply because they came from a volunteer. He can be so defensive that the board feels forced to treat him with kid gloves. Executives must be willing to give and take, to acknowledge fallibility, and to resist treating every decision as a personal vote of confidence. On occasion, the truly powerful executive directors should even be prepared to make themselves vulnerable. We teach our kids, "If you don't know, say so." In an organization, that is not necessarily executive indecisiveness, but rather good judgment.

"One of the chief things an executive director must do is to pump up the board . . . keep them excited."

ROSANN WISMAN

"The most important knack an executive director can possess in terms of the board, is to make these volunteers feel valuable."

ELAINE JACOBSON

Summary. The relationship between board and executive director is truly a partnership. The ultimate destiny of the affiliate resides with both parties. There are boundaries between their roles; after all, as Robert Frost says in "Mending Walls," "Good fences make good neighbors." Still, there must be sufficient gatekeeping as well as adequate access. If the partnership gets out of balance, it diminishes board and staff. If the partnership becomes strained, it must be repaired and rigorously maintained. If the partnership is working, the affiliate multiplies its chances for success.

CHAPTER TEN:

RECOMMENDATIONS FOR BOARD RENEWAL AND BOARD STRUCTURE

"Selected objectives for the ideal board member: know why the organization exists, and annually review why it should; give money, or help get it, or both; face budgets with courage, endowments with doubt, deficits with dismay and recover quickly from a surplus; interpret the organization's work to the public in words of two syllables; combine a New England sense of obligation with an Irish sense of humor."

MICHAEL DAVIS
Rosewald Fund

Introduction. We have not yet discussed two areas that are of great concern to contemporary nonprofit boards. The first, which I call *board renewal,* is concerned with how an affiliate gets a board and keeps it going. In other words, how does an affiliate recruit a capable, diverse board of directors, keep them inspired, connect them with the organization's history and culture, give them time to understand the organization's problems, and retain their services for long enough to reap their wisdom? A second key issue is *board structure.* How does the board structure itself so that it is able to function as an effective team and to ensure that the whole (the entire board) is bigger than the sum of its parts (typically, standing committees)?

Board renewal has three important elements: recruitment, retreat, and retention. *Recruitment* of new members, which is typically handled by the nominating committee, has become extremely challenging with changing demographics, intense competition for the very best members, and the absolute requirement that boards be ethnically diverse, balanced by experience and background, and able to succeed at the five essential board roles. *Retreat* suggests the need for boards to take time to get away from the myriad of short-term demands that compete for their attention and to spend some uninterrupted quality time with each other. In these "retreat" settings, people really get to know each other, to understand how different individuals feel and think, and to work and play with enough time to create what in the theatre is referred to as "ensemble." *Retention* is the capacity of boards to hold onto their members so that the organization can receive the "return on investment" and benefit from the wisdom that comes with experience. Keeping one's very best board members happens by making board work interesting and challenging, while at the same time not overwhelming the board with unrealistic expectations.

Renewal

Nominating the Best. Since the mid-1970s, the recruiting pool of people who might serve on Planned Parenthood boards has been drained and strained. Women have long been in the majority on Planned Parenthood boards simply because our organization's mission is so central to the lives, well-being, and equality of women. Yet with the emerging phenomenon of two-career families and single-parent families, time has become the most precious and scarce commodity for many people, especially for women. As nonprofits become more and more important to our communities (the proliferation of nonprofits is outstripping the growth in the public and private sectors), the competition for board members will become increasingly brutal as nonprofits snap up talented board members left and right. Furthermore, it has become increasingly apparent that it is essential to have a diverse board whose members represent the racial, ethnic, and cultural makeup of communities. However, for a number of reasons, minority board members may often be the hardest to recruit.

"The key to building racially and ethnically diverse boards is that the president and executive must actively build bridges into the minority community. It can be as simple as loaning space to a local group that works with black adolescents or to creating programs that combine the issues of family planning with such basic needs as teaching job skills.

The goal of diverse boards will take time

"At the onset, I provide the nominating committee an analysis by board background, gender, race, board meeting attendance—a thorough turnover analysis."

LEE MINTO

and will require patience. We can't simply get frustrated because of the reality that many organizations go after the same people. There will be false starts and mistakes will be made. But what it will do for the strenthening of the board is worth the effort."

DR. KENNETH EDELIN

These problems—fewer women with time to volunteer, more nonprofits competing for the best board members, the difficulties of finding ethnic and racial minorities for board membership—make it tough enough to find good, solid board members. Other dynamics specific to Planned Parenthood further complicate the matter. Most Planned Parenthood affiliates do not use clinic or education volunteers anymore, and that shuts down a natural recruitment pipeline. As more and more affiliates begin to merge or spread their services over hundreds of miles, it becomes more difficult for boards to recruit new members because of the extensive travel obligations and the less intimate nature of a regional board. It also may be that the controversial nature and high visibility of our issues scare off some professionals (e.g., lawyers, bankers, elected officials).

Solutions are not easy to find. However, a truly competent board in the 1990s must be composed in balanced and diverse ways. The board must be made up of persons passionately devoted to the cause; persons who are tenured veterans of the movement mixed with youthful activists ready to get started; persons who bring to the table differing professional expertise that are helpful in policy and strategy sessions; persons whose drive is finding the funds necessary for the affiliate; women and minorities whose understanding of the stakes of our clients comes from their own life experience.

"Choose your board members wisely and you will be blessed."

BRIAN O'CONNELL

Recruitment and Retention

Figure fifteen on page 111 displays the seven steps of board renewal.

Make Nomination of New Board Members an Ongoing Process. When someone terrific pops up, act at once to get him/her "on board." Affiliates that look for new members only during the couple of months before preparing the slate for the affiliate annual meeting may lose potentially stellar board members simply because when these people were ready to get involved, the nominating cycle had just finished for the year. Thus, affiliates need to structure their bylaws so that new board members can be elected year-round.

Organize the Work of the Board so That the Time Required Is Reasonable. This may mean meeting less frequently, reducing the number of committees and/or committee meetings, and consolidating board work into sessions that are less frequent but take larger blocks of time. This resembles a model of the PPFA national board or a university board of trustees, with a Friday night and full Saturday schedule. If the time requirements for a board are unrealistic and this does not get acknowledged and changed, an informal coping mechanism inevitably manifests itself: People simply start missing meetings and skipping committees. Dealing with the consequences of sporadic attendance is far more difficult than setting realistic time commitments from the start.

> ***"Board members don't always have an intuitive mystique or skills to do the job. If this is important work, then proper training must be done."***
>
> **ELAINE JACOBSON**

Provide Ongoing Training and Development Activities for the Board. One of the most powerful incentives for serving on a board is personal and professional growth. This seems especially true for younger board members who are perhaps serving on their first board. Board members often want to gain new skills and understanding, whether it is comprehending how to compute the ratio-analysis on the affiliate's net worth statement or understanding more fully how high-risk behaviors in adolescents are interconnected with teenage parenthood. Furthermore, people who choose to join affiliate boards universally hope to get some further experience in leadership thinking and behavior. A reasonable budget that allows for consultants and trainers to work with the board is money well spent.

The most critical development/training session for new board members is the orientation session. Allow your new board members to hit the ground running by orienting them right away to the strategic plan and board policies. The first three to six months is often when new

FIGURE FIFTEEN:

Recommendations for Board Renewal

I. RECRUITMENT AND RETENTION
1. Make nominating an ongoing process
2. Organize the work of the board in a reasonable time frame
3. Provide board training and development
4. Deal with controversy
   - Make issues concrete and personal
   - Understand the difference between cause and effect
   - Create support systems
5. Creatively maintain continuity

II. RETREAT
6. Organize overnight sessions
7. Pass on organizational culture, history, and pride

board members will decide to stay or leave. New board members are anxious to make a contribution to board work as quickly as possible, and if they haven't been adequately prepared, they may lose interest and gravitate elsewhere.

". . . it is important to mention there are two personal gains to which every board member is entitled. The first is personal satisfaction from assuming this role and responsibilities; the second is personal growth."

ANDREW SWANSON

Coping with Controversy. Sometimes affiliate boards have been weakened because Planned Parenthood has been so relentlessly under attack by the antichoice movement. This controversy may at times mean that an affiliate either cannot recruit certain members or won't be able to hold onto them. Without a doubt, *establishment* types can expect smoother sailing and appreciation by joining the local hospital or girl scout board. Most affiliate boards have found that it is better not to "sugar coat" the controversial nature of their work, but rather to create ongoing mechanisms to arm board members with ways to cope—in fact, ways to turn this controversial nature from a liability to an asset.

"A highly supportive board can give an organization a tremendous boost, perhaps especially an organization like Planned Parenthood which faces numerous challenges and complex, thorny issues."

***Board Papers,* written by PPFA Western Regional Office**

The best Planned Parenthood boards have adopted coping mechanisms to help members handle the controversy that comes hand-in-hand with working for Planned Parenthood. Here are three ideas.

- AVOID ABSTRACTIONS BY MAKING ISSUES CONCRETE AND PERSONAL: The best way for board members to figure out what they think about issues that are controversial is to get past the simplistic, sound-bite mentality, and get to the heart of the matter. Boards can personalize the issues by hearing

The Uniqueness of Planned Parenthood Boards:

The 1988 Survey.

Ninety percent of the executive directors felt there was something special or different about a Planned Parenthood board, as compared with other nonprofits in their communities. Almost 40 percent suggested that the biggest distinguishing factor was an extraordinary belief in the Planned Parenthood cause and mission. Twenty percent cited the level of controversy experienced by the organization as being the major differentiating factor. Other comments of special note were that Planned Parenthood boards were "working boards," that they were "held to a higher standard."

Board presidents overwhelmingly agreed. Almost 87 percent felt that serving on a Planned Parenthood board was indeed unique and different from serving on other boards. The level of controversy associated with our organization was the primary distinction; second was the necessary high degree of belief and commitment to our cause; third was the notion that Planned Parenthood boards were more sophisticated intellectually, better informed, and more professional than other boards. Interviews with board leaders confirmed that one of the key reasons behind this shared sense of board competence was that affiliates were part of a national organization, with colleagues for comparison and forums in which to learn from each other.

case studies of people in real situations, by reading letters from clients, or by talking directly with the people we work for. Rather than just debating the pros and cons of sexual abstinence for adolescents, bring in four 16-year-olds for a candid panel discussion.

- KEEP CLEAR ON THE DIFFERENCE BETWEEN CAUSE AND EFFECT: To remain true to Planned Parenthood's mission requires our affiliates to address many of the symptoms of failure in American society, including the disintegration of family, teenage drug use and promiscuity, unintended pregnancy, and this country's persistent underclass. Because we are involved with these issues, we are sometimes blamed for causing them. Planned Parenthood boards and staff must have pride in our courage and willingness to face unpopular and difficult problems.

- CREATE SUPPORT SYSTEMS EVEN BEFORE THE GOING GETS TOUGH: It is important to network with other board members and other Planned Parenthood boards when the issues become difficult or disintegrate into personal attacks by the opposition or media. Knowing you are not alone in the struggle makes continuing easier. Having a chance to practice responding to the tough questions contained in the *PPFA Issues Manual* is very helpful in gaining confidence and perspective.

The good news is that controversy and struggle magnetically attract certain individuals to our cause. Many Planned Parenthooders are always looking for a good fight if it is based on a struggle for justice and equality. Planned Parenthood's mission provides a forum for the fighters for social justice in our communities.

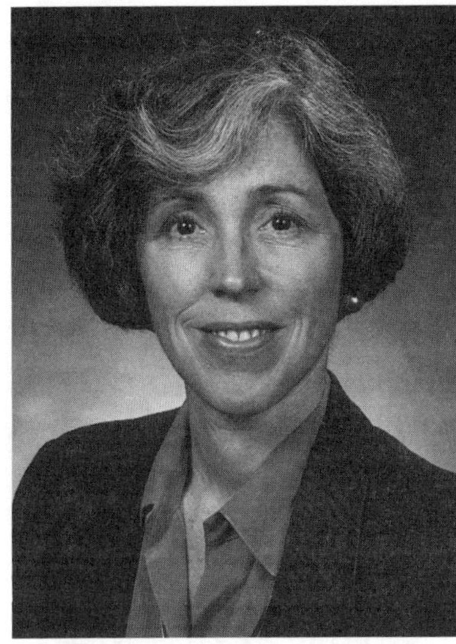

"Some board members thrive on crisis — it clarifies why they are important. But it can be hard on them when there are no 'rescue missions' needed."

SUE MOMEYER

Board Continuity: Don't Throw Out the Old Just to Bring in the New. Almost every board has some predetermined limit of office (usually six years) spelled out in its bylaws, at which point an individual cannot continue to be a member of the board. In theory, this seems a very reasonable mechanism; certainly no person is indispensable! But the underlying notion that rotation of the board eliminates deadwood is fallacious. If something is rotting, waiting for six years is ridiculous. If something is blooming, cutting it off prematurely is equally ridiculous.

Experience shows that many contemporary boards suffer more from too much turnover than from too little. In practice, busy and transient lifestyles create a substantial turnover of members leaving office before their six-year term is up. Rather than having too many long-term board members, boards can find themselves facing key decisions with too many members with an average tenure of less than a year. It can be dangerous to have a board with few members able to talk about the context of previous decisions or few who took part in historical deliberations that shaped the affiliate.

It is essential to give your board officers some latitude in the bylaws so that if their board tenure limit comes up while they are midway through serving in their leadership capacity, their term is automatically extended by virtue of their office. It can be counterproductive to lose a board president in the middle of delicate merger negotiations or a top-flight development chair halfway through a capital campaign.

"A strong board and a confident executive will insist on planned board turnover. Dead wood rots, live trees bloom."

HENRY GOLDSTEIN

Retreat

Becoming a Team. Boards need time to know each other, the opportunity to hear the tribal stories of the affiliate, and a chance to play. Board work needs to be interesting, enjoyable, and occasionally exhilarating. Certainly boards deal with serious issues, which have consequences that can be of the utmost importance. However, board meetings do not have to be so tightly organized that spontaneity is impossible. Paradoxically, in order to really confront our serious work in a meaningful way, we must ensure that there is a time for laughter and play. The time set aside for play can allow for a group volleyball game or a facilitated group creativity process exercise or performance of a skit fantasizing a conversation among George Bush, Sandra Day O'Connor, David Souter, and Clarence Thomas. These types of activities reduce the tension and avoid a paralyzing anxiety that can come when a group is too solemn and worried. Creative deliberation flourishes in groups where there is a comfortable "give and take."

"Boards spend too little time on orientation and socialization."

ETHELYN BISHOP

One of the difficulties encountered by many boards is that they do not know each other as individuals, but only as board members or as the data contained in a curriculum vitae. Boards must find ways to establish a sense of trust and professional intimacy. This bonding reduces stilted communication and establishes the all-important feeling that one is a part of a team. Without trust and confidence in each other, board members may squabble or fail to get on with the business at hand. Boards made up of people who like and respect each other soar to great heights; those that do not, dive for safe perches. The following techniques help to create a sense of community or team.

Organize Overnight Sessions. These are overnights where the board has an opportunity to break bread and sip wine with one another. Often, at these occasions, the board is given the rare privilege to focus on just a few important themes. It is helpful to provide an outside facilitator who can offer some fresh perspectives and manage the event so that all the members (especially the president) are free to participate. In addition, the event should be organized so that it focuses on the future; in this way the board's time together is really a board "advance" rather than a "retreat." In other words, the board is getting away from the daily details of operational demands so that it can look out onto the horizon and choose paths to advance the affiliate toward success and health.

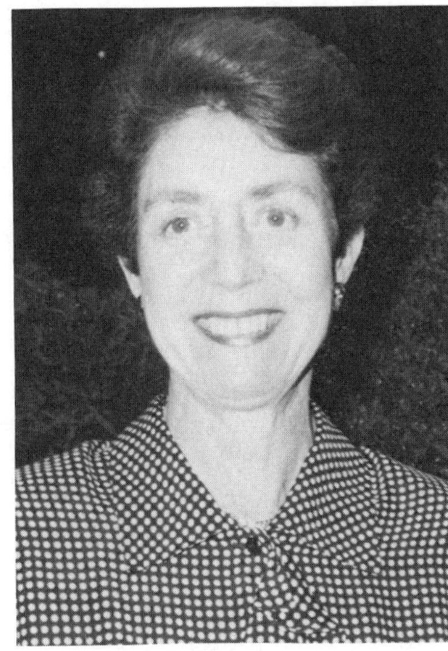

"Make sure the board gets a chance to decide on issues that really mean something. A feeling of being on the inside . . ."

ELAINE JACOBSON

Pass on the Organization's Culture, History, and Pride from One Board Generation to Another. Nothing bonds a new board member to the affiliate like hearing the story of an inspiring moment in an affiliate's history. Sitting in a comfortable room while board old-timers reminisce about the best and worst times in the affiliate's history can lead to some powerful and magical moments. "Remember the day we locked arms when the rescue fanatics rushed our clinic's front door . . . remember when we burned the mortgage on our downtown office . . . remember the board meeting right after the Webster decision when we just sat in silence for five minutes?" Hearing these kinds of anecdotes of an affiliate's oral history will give a new board member a context, a historical perspective, and a sense of belonging in a powerful and dramatic way. But it requires the board to give itself the time to truly get away from it all.

Structure

Organizing the Board's Work. Boards often divide their members and tasks into committees. In theory, committees are designed to make the work of the board manageable and more efficient. The concept is to have a small group of board members focus on a particular part of the agency's work, such as budget and finance, thereby relieving the full board from having to understand every aspect of the affiliate's financial operations. Unfortunately, it is hard to find affiliates where a majority of its board committees seem to contribute on a cost-to-contribution basis. At best, they often take too much time and energy; at worst, they leave the full board completely out of pertinent discussion. Here are common complaints about committees:

- Committee attendance is sporadic, and getting any sense of continuity on tasks that require multiple meetings is virtually impossible.

- Committees get peopled with non-board members, so sometimes when their work advances to the board, a majority of the committee is not present to share the thinking of their proposals.
- Committees engage in the most intriguing policy deliberations, often leaving the full board out of interesting discussions and leaving them with no alternative but to rubber stamp the committee's recommendations.
- Committees traditionally are constructed to parallel the important program and administrative functions of the agency, resulting in an invitation for meddling or redundancy. For instance, in the past decade marketing has become vital to many affiliates' abilities to offer competitive, consumer-centered reproductive health services. Thus, some affiliates have created marketing committees on their board. If, however, a board has committed itself to dealing primarily at the strategic planning and policy level, as I am recommending in this book, then working at the operational level of marketing is not in the board's domain.
- Committee support requires much time and energy from staff. As the marginal sidebar shows, in my 1988 survey, staff reported spending a considerable amount of time on work relating to board committees. It is impossible by simple mathematics to figure out whether the staff cost for support of committees is too much or too little. It completely depends upon whether the committee work adds value to the yield of the board product (i.e., good decisions leading to affiliate success). But, clearly, staff involvement does have a discrete, calculable expense, and this expense can be significant. On that basis alone, it is vital to spend the right amount of time and to spend the time right.

> **Committees:**
>
> *The 1988 Survey.*
>
> According to the baseline data established in the survey, executive directors attended over 75 percent of the board committee meetings. At the same time, a number of executive directors interviewed gave the impression that some of these committees were unnecessary and ineffective. If that is so, then the significant amount of time executive directors spend with committees should be questioned. Executives spend almost 70 hours a year at committee meetings. If one uses a conservative estimate that for every hour spent in the actual meeting, it requires another two hours in preparation, follow-up, and travel, then the executive spends more than 200 hours a year on committee meetings, or a whopping 10 percent of his or her time. And the executive director's time is only a partial accounting of staff costs for committee work. Many affiliates have other senior staff beyond the executive director routinely attend meetings, estimated by some to average somewhere close to the equivalent of one full-time person. Since the staff who attend committee and board meetings are in senior positions, their salaries are the highest in the agency, adding to the expense of the committee process.

Organizing Committees to Succeed. Each affiliate board must reconsider its committees, and pare them down to the essentials. Some typical approaches are:

- Give committees a clear, understandable, and doable charge.
- Hold committee meetings in concert with (before or after) board meetings so that travel time is minimized.
- Reduce the number of committees from twelve, which was the affiliate average found in the survey, to no more than absolutely required (six?). Make sure that committees do not parallel staff program and administration functions, but rather correspond to *board* roles and responsibilities. For example, the board's work in long-range planning could be accomplished by a long-range plan-

ning committee. The board's fiduciary responsibility could be carried out by the board's budget and finance committee. The board's need to sustain itself could be accomplished through a nominating committee.

- Eliminate or consolidate administrative committees, such as personnel, budget, and investment.
- Eliminate most standing committees in favor of short-term task forces or "ad hoc" work groups that can respond to critical new ventures that are short-term needs, such as mergers and capital campaigns. When their job is done, eliminate them.
- Write in an abbreviated style committee minutes that are distributed to board to provide an executive summary of actions taken or areas in which new board policies are recommended. This gives the board a helpful tool to get quickly to the essence of committee deliberation.
- Separate some traditional committees from the province of the board, making them directly responsible to staff for general advisory purposes. For example, it is my opinion that affiliate medical committees are not subsets of the board. Rather, medical committees are advisory groups for medical staff. The medical committee's role is to consult with the medical director so that affiliate clinical practices are congruent with accepted community medical standards. The implication here is that affiliate boards that structure themselves with medical committees as board committees have followed a logic which would require them to review all of the medical committee's work and ratify all of their decisions. No affiliate board has the time or expertise to exercise this kind of control.

> ***"A committee is a group that keeps minutes and loses hours."***
>
> **MILTON BERLE**

Conclusion. The two essential points captured in this chapter are that boards need the most talented members they can find and then need to organize themselves in a simple fashion to be both efficient and effective. The first point is *renewal*—the ability to recruit diverse and committed members to replace old members, the commitment to retain those individuals who are outstanding, and the need to give board members ample opportunity to replenish themselves in frequent retreats. The second point is *structure*—the need to structure the board's work by keeping things simple, avoiding an overabundance of committees and operating in such a way that the action stays at the board level. The more complex the structure, the more bureaucratic the pace. Boards that create lively work processes and simple organizing structures are far more likely to feel good about themselves and to do good work.

CHAPTER ELEVEN:

MAKING A GOOD BOARD GREAT:

The Importance of Taking Risks Wisely

Successful Affiliates Create Successful Boards—and Vice Versa. Board success does not come simply from fancy technique at running tight meetings or even from knowing how to plan for the future. Rather, good boards almost always are found in affiliates that are running terrific programs, attracting talented staff, and, just as often as not, exceeding their goals.

> *"Eliminate risk and you eliminate innovation . . . in a plan, don't eliminate risk; knowingly take it on."*
>
> VAUGHN KELLER

> ***"No pain, no gain. No attempt, no triumph. No disappointment, no achievement. No cross, no crown."***
>
> **JEROLD PANAS**

How do all these good things happen? The crucial variable seems to be that great outcomes spring from the organization's willingness to take risks. The most critical difference between an average board and a great board is not the board's way of doing work but the willingness to take risks, to innovate, to become obsessed with the concerns of the Planned Parenthood movement.

"Boards may only confront an affiliate-shaping decision but once a year. Yet when it happens they must be prepared to act."

ROSANN WISMAN

Success Requires Risk. Powerful affiliates, both large and small, that are visionary risk takers understand the essential dynamic of risk. Unfortunately, the concept of risk has been stuck with a negative connotation. It is true that risk taking does involve uncertainty. Embarking upon unknown territory is uncomfortable. No one guaranteed the board of Syracuse Planned Parenthood that providing outpatient abortion services would work in 1973; or Planned Parenthood of New York City that bold advocacy ads could really influence public opinion; or Rocky Mountain Planned Parenthood that family planning could be run as a business. But what a loss it would have been for the entire movement if these boards had not taken the opportunity to test these innovations. These boards realized that to break new ground required risk. They also understood that risk must be undertaken with a thorough understanding of what the organization is and what it stands for.

As a capitalist or social revolutionary knows, the greater the risk, the greater the payoff—if one is successful. Thus, John Paul Getty and Margaret Sanger understood that the risk taker tries to navigate around the perils of loss and uncertainty and land the profitable gain of big ideas and bold ventures. *The profit for an affiliate is not money, but breakthrough programs that make a quantum leap towards the accomplishment of its mission.*

"The highest use of capital is not to make more money, but to make money do more for the betterment of life."

HENRY FORD

"Boards must avoid 'analysis paralysis' when it comes to making decisions. Tom Peters' bromide must be remembered (namely, it is sometimes better to) fire, ready, aim . . . than worry about each shot."

NORAH HOLMGREN

Three Different Paths. It is said that a board tends to operate primarily in one of three ways—as a caretaker, a risk taker, or an undertaker. The CARETAKER board avoids major errors or mistakes. Board members monitor activities to make sure adequate programmatic and administrative competence is achieved. They exert just enough stewardship to ensure that the organization they inherited from their predecessors is roughly equivalent to the one they will pass on to their successors.

"Boards can't drift, but must change. What is most critical at a given point in time is directed by the shape of major events."

FAYE WATTLETON

The RISK TAKER board understands that risk is the price paid for progress, growth, and expansion; that adequate financial capital is the coin necessary to strike out in new directions; and that bold transformational leadership is a minimum requirement. These risk takers want to be remembered as a group of policy-making strategists who seized opportunity while simultaneously vanquishing threats. They want to be remembered not just for defending the mission, but also for striving to make the affiliate better and stronger for the future. The risk taker board is like a giraffe: "one who sticks his neck out for the common good!" A risk-taking board is willing to consider changes such as expansion, new programs, mergers, and capital campaigns—all significant endeavors with no guarantees of success.

The UNDERTAKER board does not actually set out to put the affiliate six feet under, but its actions (and often inaction) are ponderous and muddled. These boards do not sustain a vision that makes an affiliate a lively place in the present or in the future. Sometimes these boards oversee organizations in visible crisis or downright shambles. The most dangerous undertaker boards run what organizational consultant George Ordione calls the "well-run bankruptcy" agency, otherwise known as an organization where "the lights are on, but nobody is home." It is these lifeless organizations that cause so much surprise and shock when they suddenly go belly-up. But the sad fact is that sometimes the organizations have been dying for years and have simply succumbed to the first serious crisis.

When confronted with these three radically different paths to the future, it becomes clear that how boards deal with risk can have life and death consequences for the health of the affiliate. Depending upon the approach taken, the affiliate can flourish as a risk taker *or* it can live a careful existence of safety at all costs, *or,* sadly, it can die. The track record is like a bell-shaped curve. Most boards operate in the middle, while only a few operate at either edge, exhibiting excellence or deadly incompetence.

Stakes Too High to Duck Risk. Many boards set out with a sincere desire to make a positive and lasting contribution. However, most boards also secretly dread the worst case scenario that somehow they will be in charge when the affiliate is placed in receivership with a Chapter 11 bankruptcy or is decertified by the Federation. Because a majority of boards seek success while struggling to fend off defeat, they end up settling for the caretaking middle ground. Thus they spend most of their time playing it safe, doing everything in moderation.

Unfortunately, this middle ground has really never been all that safe and sure. Instead, it is actually often the edge of a slippery slope. In this turbulent era of the early 1990s, middle-of-the-road leadership usually means sliding into the abyss of mediocrity and attempting the frustrating approach of being all things to everyone.

The threats to Planned Parenthood affiliates in the 1990s will likely be more perilous than anything we have seen in the last 75 years. Our buildings have been attacked with terrorist bombs, and our patients come to us both poorer and sicker. The last two United States presidential administrations have attempted to destroy our funding and our resolve. In this climate, boards must undertake the risks necessary to keep the banner flying proudly and high.

Some family planning organizations look at this turbulence and arrive at the conclusion that the way to cope is to become very careful and exceedingly cautious. Their boards ask very safe questions. Maybe we can appease the Department of Health and Human Services by following the guidance of the "gag rule"? Maybe we can steer clear of the potential wrath of the local health maintenance organization if we don't advertise for clients? Maybe we should remain quiet about an openly anti-choice Supreme Court nominee, so that we don't alienate our most conservative donors? These are all legitimate questions, and in the short-term, conservative responses would be less risky. But like the national organization founded by Margaret Sanger, most Planned Parenthood affiliates have found that saying "no" to playing it safe is a risk that in the long term is well worth taking. For in the reproductive health movement, the legacy for Planned Parenthood is to be on the cutting edge, and to finish the agenda that Sanger drew up 75 years ago.

> ***"Boards sometimes are overconcerned with a fear of failure. A successful board has enough resources to make a few mistakes."***
>
> **ETHELYN BISHOP**

Managing Risk. Risk does not mean willy-nilly gambling with hard-earned assets, such as financial well-being or the good name and reputation of Planned Parenthood. Boards must fulfill their legal responsibilities, including the duties of care, loyalty, obedience, and diligence (discussed in Chapter Three). As experienced Planned Parenthood leaders have learned in developing medical quality assurance programs and setting up our captive insurance company, risk can and must be *managed.* If PPFA had not set up the wholly owned Planned Protection Insurance Company (PPIC) in 1977, there would not be the affiliate development that we witness over 15 years later. Affiliate budgets would have been drained by higher premium payments; national office time would have been diverted to plugging holes in a spotty and hemorrhaging commercial insurance industry. Like any management activity, risk must be planned comprehensively, implemented carefully, and monitored frequently. The following approaches are prudent ways to approach risk:

- SPREAD THE RISK AROUND. Affiliates should never put their entire operations on the line or all their eggs in one basket. The best way to make big changes without taking big chances is to have a broad mixture of funding, kinds of programs, and types of clients. The ideal diversity might be achieving significant funding streams in the three areas that have historically underwritten our services—government grants, patient fees, and private fund raising. Programmatic balance would come from multiple types of medical services provided—contraception, infertility, prenatal, abortion. Creating a balanced array of client types could be achieved by broadening the dimension on any number of demographic fronts—low and middle income, urban and suburban, adolescents and peri-menopausal women. The point is that it is easier to risk making a possible mistake when its effect would be reduced because the organization still has other funds/programs/clients to turn to. Affiliates should only undertake riskier new ventures if they can maintain their dependable bread-and-butter programs.

- SELECT RISK STRATEGICALLY. When affiliates choose new endeavors that have a degree of risk, they should take these chances only on activities that, if they are successful, pay handsome dividends financially or make headway towards mission achievement. To undertake risk for a tangential goal is foolish. Those nonprofits that have gone too deeply into unrelated business pursuits, ostensibly to make a handsome profit, but have then seen the deal fail, provide a striking reminder of what to avoid.

- PREPARE FOR RISK. Affiliates that take risks must have viable contingency plans if things do not work out. The best safety nets are having money in the bank and a "reserve" of good will in the community. Sound advice for Planned Parenthood affiliates is to consider taking risks in *program* while being conservative *financially.* This often means acquiring and retiring adequate reserve funding to provide a soft landing in the event of failure, and having clearly defined escape routes if the new venture flounders. In other words, if an affiliate has salted away a million dollars in the bank, the risk of investing $250,000 in a new clinic does not put the affiliate in jeopardy. However, an affiliate with just a quarter of a million dollars in its fund balance would be taking an enormous chance contemplating that very same clinic expansion. The statistical probability on taking risks is irrefutable; a certain percentage of the time, one will fail.

- SHARE RISKS. Affiliates should find partners who will carry some of the burden if the risk fails. This can mean seeking outside funders or crafting joint ventures with other affiliates, nonprofits, or the private sector. In late 1991, Planned Parenthoods in Los Angeles and Denver joined together to purchase national direct mail lists, the cost of which to either affiliate alone would have been prohibitive. As another example, an affiliate that is considering placing a new clinic close to several large factories might ask each company to chip in $50,000 for start-up expenditures. The companies could see this as beneficial if they are concerned about keeping a work force of healthy women. The affiliate could see this partnership as advantageous because it would both minimize the need to use affiliate funds in start-up and create a vested interest by the companies in the success of the clinic.

- UNDERSTAND AND SUPPORT RISK. Any affiliate looking at a new, risky venture should clearly understand the potential upside and downside. Once the risk is understood, affiliate leadership must stand by a collective decision; should the venture fail, it will do no good to lay blame on one individual or group.

If managed correctly, a Planned Parenthood need never fail to do the right thing simply because to do it would expose the affiliate to some risk. Imagine what a liberated feeling it would be if every Planned Parenthood board could always do what it felt was right because it had deployed a sufficient number of fail-safe mechanisms—multiple locations, diversified patient loads, adequate reserves, risk-sharing partners—that would ensure against affiliate failure if things went badly. The strength of each affiliate having a broader "shield of contingencies" would accelerate the pace of growth, expansion, and development throughout the entire federation.

Risk: A Way of Life for Planned Parenthood. If risk is present in all nonprofits, it is doubly true for Planned Parenthood. Directing a Planned Parenthood affiliate is seldom simple, safe, or static. If we are doing what we are supposed to be doing, we are CHANGE AGENTS, taking on the good fight for the silent majority that supports our efforts but often avoids the controversy of it all. When one's mission demands speaking and acting for the disenfranchised, engaging in the arena of sexual politics, and fighting for the rights of women and men to take responsibility for their reproductive lives, risk-taking goes with the territory. Things might have gone more smoothly if Planned Parenthood had kept quiet on the "squeal rule," but patient care for adolescents would have been compromised. It might have been more congruent to our bipartisan "roots" if Planned Parenthood hadn't joined the fight against the confirmation of Robert Bork to the Supreme Court, but privacy protections would have fared worse. It is often easier not to provide abortion care, but patients want that choice available without having to be referred out the door.

If we become just a part of the health care delivery system or a quasi-governmental agency, even if we perform in an exemplary way, then we are failing our purpose of making "every child a wanted child." Occasionally challenging a traditional funding source, confronting the assumptions of the local medical establishment, or taking on unpopular political battles goes with the territory of social change.

Problems in the '90s That Create a Moral Imperative to Take Risks Wisely. Often when discussion involves central values and the abstract ideas of risk, the concepts sound so good that board members will nod their heads in agreement. However, when the organization needs to decide on specifics, too often boards back off and executives look the other way. Our federation of affiliates loses ground when our actual behavior and accomplishments don't parallel the values we endorse. Although we have claimed huge victories in the last decade, and rightly so, there are also a set of vulnerabilities that individually and collectively we cannot tolerate if we are to succeed in the 1990s. This federation needs the affiliates and national office to find the time, money, energy, and common cause to address some big gaps in our capacity to succeed. We need to take the risk to talk to each other, not *at* each other. We need to provide the risk capital to enable the consolidation of affiliates with full spectrum medical services, and comprehensive education services, and political programs strong enough to strike fear in the hearts of our opposition.

Planned Parenthood in Vermont:

RISKING LEGISLATURE DEFUNDING AND LIVING TO TELL ABOUT IT

Setting the Stage. In 1978, the board of Planned Parenthood of Vermont (PPV)* decided that women in one of the communities it served needed access to a safe and affordable abortion service. The board made a policy decision that the continuum of reproductive health care should include this new service. The executive director prepared an acceptable business plan and the service began. The uproar and pressures that the affiliate faced over the next 18 months tested the board's resolve, its group problem-solving skills, its ability to share leadership with the executive director, and its capacity to make a far-reaching decision that involved taking a considerable risk.

The Legislature Convenes. In February of 1979, Planned Parenthood of Vermont, as a delegate agency of the Vermont Health Department, had been awarded a research grant from the Department of Health and Human Services (DHHS) to study rural family planning issues. The Vermont legislature was just starting its legislative session. One of its first chores was the rather boring and technical practice of passing a supplemental budget appropriation, which this year included the Planned Parenthood grant.

During this supplemental budget process, an outspoken anti-choice state senator became aware that PPV had begun providing privately funded abortion services; PPV had performed 52 abortion procedures at its Rutland clinic in the start-up year of 1978.

This senator moved to block the research grant for PPV—although it had nothing to do with the abortion service—with vitriolic accusations and mean-sounding rhetoric. For weeks, the story was front-page news. With all the media attention and the false impressions spawned by 30-second sound bites, the PPV board received bi-weekly updates on what was happening. Fortunately, the Vermont Senate overrode his objections, mostly on the technical grounds that this project was already under way and that a research project was not the proper subject for contesting the issue.

OBSERVATION: Keep the board informed: When havoc breaks out, boards need frequent information to stay abreast of a rapidly changing situation.

However, the Senator's action gave anti-choice forces the go-ahead to begin a serious attack on the affiliate. On the final day of the 1979 legislative session, a second anti-abortion senator concocted another resolution. His argument was this: It was a conflict of interest for PPV, the state's family planning provider, to

* PPV was the predecessor affiliate of Planned Parenthood of Northern New England (PPNNE). PPV was a state-wide affiliate serving all of Vermont. In 1984 the affiliate merged with the Upper Valley Planned Parenthood affiliate in New Hampshire and in 1991 merged with a family planning agency in southern Maine. PPNNE is now a three-state affiliate.

attempt to prevent the need for abortion while doing abortions at the same time. The new resolution threatened to take away all federal and state family planning dollars if PPV did not stop providing abortion services. A group of PPV board members who knew Lieutenant Governor Madeleine Kunin as a friend and political confidante met with her within the first week of the crisis to give her the facts of the situation. The Senate vote was 15-15, but the Lieutenant Governor broke the tie in the affiliate's favor. Unfortunately, this setback was seen as only momentary by the opposition. In the Senate chamber, anti-choice senators quickly held a press conference to say that PPV had better obey their cease-and-desist order or the anti-choicers would get the votes to make the resolution stick when the Senate reconvened eight months later.

OBSERVATION: Board connections help in the political arena. Political and media events move swiftly. It is crucial that Planned Parenthood supporters (often its board) have solid experience in their public affairs role, in order to have access to the halls of political power when the need arises.

The Grim Situation. This defunding attempt was a very serious threat. In 1979, government-related funds made up 91 percent of PPV's budget. PPV was the entire family planning program in Vermont (every clinic in the state was operated by the affiliate) and the exclusive recipient of Title X funding. Over 80 percent of the program was basic contraceptive services and community education. Throughout the state, particularly in rural areas, PPV provided the only health care people received, and if PPV was not there, they would not get *any* primary health care. The agency's budget was $800,000, but no more than $37,000 had ever been raised privately. PPV was way too heavy in government grants and way too light in fund raising. Public affairs efforts were handled solely by the board Information and Education Committee and a half-time public information coordinator.

The financial implications placed the board in a very difficult spot. Could the board place the entire organization in jeopardy for this brand new and minuscule abortion service? What would happen to the 12,000 family planning patients who would suffer dire consequences if PPV were put out of existence? At this point enemies in the legislature seemed determined to make PPV retreat or surrender. Even worse, many of the affiliate's best friends—legislators, public officials, donors—felt that compromise was the only way to go. PPV was told over and over again that the anti-choice legislators would likely win in 1980 and that the pragmatic course of action would be a hasty retreat for the greater good of protecting essential family planning services.

All the other demands of the world didn't go away just because the PPV board had big trouble in one arena. As if this crisis weren't enough, the PPV board had just voted to relocate the administrative office and main clinic by renovating an old Red Cross Blood Bank building into a modern facility. It needed to raise $500,000 in capital funds to do this. In fact, the agency had already bought the building, gotten a short-term mortgage for interim financing, and signed the construction contract—all with only 20 percent of the needed money raised, pledged, or even in sight.

OBSERVATION: Boards that take risks must operate on many fronts simultaneously. In order to accomplish this, they need to split up the work (i.e., task forces) and expect quality staff work. They must keep moving forward the projects they have already begun.

Slow Down and Study. The statewide

media were hounding the agency to announce its decision. Everyone assumed an immediate decision by PPV was the only way to control the damage. The board's first decision, however, was not to do anything in haste. The president set up a task force to work for three months to develop a series of recommendations for the full board to consider in the fall of 1979. Their charge was to analyze the four most apparent options: (1) explore litigation on federal statutory grounds, should the anti-choice lawmakers prevail; (2) test the feasibility of counter-legislation; (3) reduce expenses and increase fees in existing affiliate programs; and (4) develop new programs financed with private sources, not government funds.

Over the summer months, the six-person task force, along with the executive director and president, sifted through masses of data and various alternatives and contingency reports prepared by the staff. Ultimately this task force came to realize that this issue was one of conviction, not of fancy, complicated solutions. Simply put, the agency's fundamental mission was at risk. Although there were strategies that would mitigate the agency's complete financial destruction, there was no foolproof way out of the crisis. If the anti-choice forces were able to get the votes they needed, the agency would immediately be halved in size and would be forced to lay off capable staff and eliminate good programs. The task force came to a rather stark conclusion: either back down immediately or engage in a fight in which losing could have both painful and damaging consequences.

Preparing for the Decision Point. As the September meeting drew closer, the board president and executive director realized that the entire board needed to participate fully in this decision. To accomplish this, a consultant would be hired to facilitate the meeting. The executive director sought out someone who understood the abortion issue and who respected the integrity of the board's dual responsibility to make its own decision and to then prepare for the consequences of that decision. Fortunately, it was the same person who had worked with staff earlier in the summer to help staff deal with their own anxiety, understand the complexity of the issue, and trust that the board would make the right decision.

The big decision board meeting drew 100 percent attendance. Everyone arrived well-briefed with the task force briefing papers. Initially, everyone appeared to be undecided. The board members seemed to know instinctively that the issue needed to be decided as a group and that to have shown up with a mind made up would have been a mistake. The staff and task force members presented their reports. The board quickly grasped the alternatives and the simple fact that, sometime late in the meeting, the buck would stop with it.

The facilitator created a process that started with facts, while allowing plenty of time for the expression of feelings. Members were encouraged to look at the big picture before prematurely leaping to a specific position. The board was divided into three theoretical Planned Parenthoods of Vermont. Each group had one of the following preassigned positions: to fight, to flee, or to straddle. The job of each group within the next two hours, was to defend, realistically, the correctness of its position and to report its game plan to the whole board.

Group One was composed of the "Fighters." Their assignment was to spit right back in the anti-choice group's eye, declare there was no retreat from principle, and instantly build the affiliate as a lean and mean political machine. Group Two, whose role was to flee, would give up the abortion service because it threatened the totality of the prevention work that the affiliate had built over 13 years. And Group Three, the straddling "Middle-of-the-Roaders," would not throw in the towel from the start, but if and when funding was taken away, would give in and announce the regrettable need to close the abortion service.

OBSERVATION: The best board deliberations include hearing all sides. The ultimate decision will be stronger if the downsides, and what turn out to be minority opinions, are fully explored.

The role-playing process proved most useful because it gave the board a chance to listen to itself. All the pros and cons were placed in the open and were passionately championed as the *RIGHT* thing to do. Even though emotions ran high and the stakes even higher, people listened and heard different points of view. Six hours of meeting time allowed most of the dimensions of the issues to be addressed and understood.

Everyone present braced themselves for the first real sign of how the board would vote. Right before a midday break, a straw vote was taken. It was meant not to be binding, but would allow the leadership to figure out what subjects needed the most time for discussion after lunch. The board members were asked to choose which of the three scenarios they supported. Twenty-two members voted to fight, one voted to stay in the middle of the road, and no one voted to flee.

OBSERVATION: By testing the waters, the chair can minimize circular conversations. Discussions on important subjects can go on forever. As long as the straw vote device is not used prematurely, it gives direction to the presiding officer.

The afternoon session gave the board the time necessary to flesh out the consequences of not backing down from the legislature. How would they build a real advocacy and lobbying program, accelerate the capital campaign and private fund raising, and increase patient fees? Board members realized that voting to defend the crucial principles at stake was not enough. They needed concurrently to address the pragmatic and business demands that would be placed upon an affiliate committed to such a risky path. Staff spelled out in broad strokes how that could be accomplished now that a tentative strategy was in place.

With the principles well articulated and the consequences spelled out in no uncertain terms, the motion to maintain abortion services was moved and seconded. The vote was unanimous, and the relief of board members was obvious. The hard work of debating the rights of the patients, the ideas of staff, and the threats of funders had been accomplished, thoroughly and well. All voices had been heard. The realities of what the decision meant had been assimilated.

OBSERVATION: Board policy-making must be informed by matters of practical feasibility. When a major decision affects the "shared domain" of board and staff, the board needs to hear from the executive director and other key staff to know the practical implications of the decision.

Subsequent events turned out to be difficult, but they were eventually as satisfying as making the board decision. The Vermont Senate, true to most predictions, voted 17-13 to take away Planned Parenthood's state and federal funding. Attention swung to the House, which was altogether untested on the abortion issue. Lobbying had been intense on both sides. Newspaper polls showed a close vote, with a majority of representatives still undecided on the day of the vote. The vote was by roll call, with activists on both sides tallying the votes as the process unfolded. Three-quarters of the way through the roll

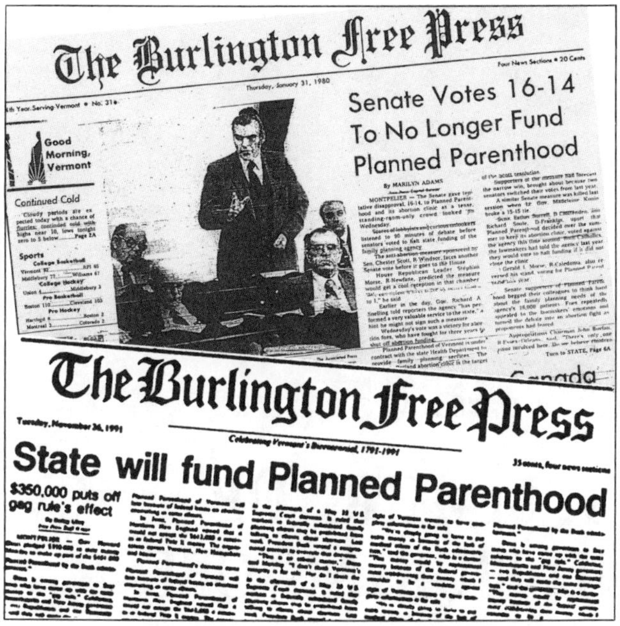

The Burlington Free Press

Senate Votes 16-14 To No Longer Fund Planned Parenthood

Good Morning, Vermont

The Burlington Free Press

State will fund Planned Parenthood

$350,000 puts off gag rule's effect

These two headlines underscore what a difference twelve years can make. PPNNE leaders are convinced that taking the risk to fight in 1980 led to the political success of 1992.

call, the resolution was defeated. Supporters of the affiliate cheered and mobbed each other in the House gallery.

Although the immediate threat was over, the affiliate also realized that the board strategy of strong advocacy and financial self-sufficiency was not a short-term tactical matter, but rather a strategic game plan that would take many years to implement. And the board members now knew that they—not a state government agency, not even well-meaning friends—were indeed the real long-term trustees of PPV's future.

OBSERVATION: Risk-taking provides boards with the single most important opportunity to make a difference. When there are no right answers and the rights of Planned Parenthood constituents are in jeopardy, the board must make judgments.

Postscript. The Vermont story exemplifies the three roles (caretaker, risk-taker, undertaker) that a board could have chosen when the legislature pushed the affiliate to the brink. Especially compelling was the safety of the middle ground. Compromising (e.g., giving up the tiny abortion service) would have been eminently rational and justifiable; all organizations face minor setbacks from time to time.

But the Vermont board correctly identified that this wasn't a case of giving a little ground in order to recapture it later, but rather a threat to the fundamental mission of the affiliate. If PPV truly believed that its central purpose was "to allow individuals to decide when, and if, to bear children," then how could the organization back down from such a core principle? The anti-choice strategy was that all-too-familiar ploy to play off preventive family planning against abortion services. What the Vermont board discovered was that these services and freedoms were not divisible.

Looking back twelve years after the decision, it is hard to know for sure what would have happened if the board had decided differently. What would the organization look like? Who would be attracted to the board? What services would it provide to its clients? What kind of fund-raising success would it enjoy?

The facts are that PPNNE has become the fifth largest affiliate in the federation, spans three states, and offers a diversified mixture of reproductive health services (including four clinics that offer abortion services). And in 1992, the Vermont legislature, in the midst of a horrible state budget crisis, became the first state lawmaking body in the country to actually appropriate additional state dollars to replace the anticipated loss of Title X funds because of the gag rule. Vermont lawmakers understood clearly (by a 2-to-1 margin) that this was simply another variation on the theme to chip away at abortion rights under the guise of restricting funding for family planning. It may be that they remember the fight and the outcome of what happened twelve years before.

AFTERWORD:

SUMMING UP AND SIGNING OFF

"The board of trustees acts to promote the mission of the organization. The trustees guarantee that the principles articulated in the mission will be carried into action."

VAUGHN KELLER

Looking Back. I began with the ambitious goal of trying to provide an overview of how Planned Parenthood boards should guide their affiliates. I have attempted to describe what this new vision of governance entails, what it requires board members to do, and conversely, what practices of boards must be given up.

I've offered concrete descriptions of board roles, responsibilities, and duties. I've presented ways to plan strategically, set corporate policy, and be a competent boss to the chief executive officer. The book has discussed how the leadership of the board (the president) can be effective and how the leadership of the affiliate (the president and the executive director) can create a working partnership. I've framed the critical dynamics of board renewal (recruitment, retreat, retention) and the most common mistakes of board structure (e.g., too many unfocused committees). Proven approaches to organizing fund raising and public policy work have been presented. I conclude by suggesting that the very best affiliate boards are those that perform the basics well and transcend the ordinary by innovating and taking risks wisely.

This view of governance is certainly not meant to be regimented; it is not a recipe that each and every affiliate should follow exactly. Certainly some affiliates have successful boards that handle many of the subject areas differently from what I propose. And since affiliates come in all shapes and forms, the ways in which their boards govern will sometimes look and feel different. But my sense is that there are several common practices that are shared by our very best boards. These very best boards don't micro-manage the affiliate's operations. They use their time well, possess a thoughtful set of values and policies, do creative long-range planning, employ a first-rate executive director, believe in the board deliberative process, find the best possible people to serve, and risk innovation and change.

"The best executive directors exert leadership by planting seeds, not by giving directives to their boards."

ANNE SAUNIER

How to Start Reinventing the Board. If this book has suggested new possibilities for the board you know best, the leadership imperative is to make the changes that most appeal to you and your organization, the changes that are of the highest priority. Some boards might choose to make wholesale changes; some boards may not so much adopt the vision of governance described in this book as carefully stop some of their current ways of operating; some boards may simply want to use a section (e.g., strategic planning), see how that works, and go accordingly from there.

But redesigning and redirecting the role of the board is difficult and risky work. It is *difficult* because no one source can help individual affiliates completely. Many affiliates are confronting major programmatic or financial challenges that require the board's unyielding attention. A board cannot take a yearlong sabbatical from its current obligations to redesign itself. The process is *risky* because it takes a confident, mature group of people to be able to exchange the status quo for the unfamiliar and to face major problems squarely while not being overwhelmed.

It is also *difficult and risky* because the board must do all this work primarily by itself and for itself. The retooling of the board *cannot* come primarily from the executive director, because the board is her superior and in the final analysis, she can't dictate to her boss. Nevertheless, the executive director does have an important role in re-creating the board. The executive director must encourage, cooperate, and enthusiastically welcome new approaches.

Fundamental board change *cannot* be dictated by external consultants because outsiders can't appreciate totally the unique demands of a Planned Parenthood organization. The redesign of governance is the unique territory of the board itself. In the final analysis, the board is in the best position to know what to fix and what not to touch. As we all know, if you fix it yourself, you own it for life.

Signing off. I love boards. Especially those in Planned Parenthood. My favorite day as an affiliate executive director is board meeting day, a day of decisions that have an impact on the future of the affiliate. My second favorite day is the day after the board meeting, a day of rest, because a successful board meeting is the hardest work that a C.E.O. encounters.

I've had the chance to meet many other affiliate board members by leading training workshops and facilitating strategic planning sessions and merger negotiations. I've seen boards in the best of times and in the throes of crisis. I've seen timid boards and brave boards. I've been convinced by at least twenty boards that they alone have to operate in the most conservative community in the United States.

What I find over and over again is that Planned Parenthood boards attract some of the most talented, intelligent, and passionate people imaginable. The same can be said for Planned Parenthood staff, but that's another book. I am continuously amazed at the caliber of fiduciaries who are attracted to our boards. Don't they know that the most powerful church in the world is willing to spend a cool $5 million to knock us out? Don't they know that the federal administration in Washington hasn't liked us for the last decade?

They *do* know, and that is why they come forward and why they come back.

My objective in sharing what I've learned about boards has been to help make sure that the talent, the intelligence, and the passion of such people can be put to the best use on a board of directors. We cannot afford to check those resources at the door. I've tried to say that there are things boards must do and things they should never do. I hope I've made the benefits of change seem worth the trouble. To board members, I say: May your plans be strategic, your policies clear, your advocacy courageous, and your fund-raising campaigns over the top. To my executive director colleagues, I say: May your boss be demanding, but fair.

ACKNOWLEDGMENTS

The list of those to whom I am indebted for assistance with this project is long and probably incomplete. I must begin with Jane Johnson and Marilyn Bowie of the national office, who believed in a contemporary book about Planned Parenthood boards and provided support to make it happen. I am grateful to the board presidents and executive directors I interviewed and who shared their insights on the art and science of boardsmanship. Their perceptive comments are quoted and interspersed throughout this book. I certainly didn't get a chance to talk to everyone who has become wise in the ways of boards. Still, no one could argue with the credentials of this illustrious crew: Faye Wattleton, Ken Edelin, and Anne Saunier, offering a national perspective; current and past board presidents, Ethelyn Bishop from Washington, D.C., Elaine Jacobson from Westchester County, New York, and Cathy Frank from Northern New England, who shared the lessons they had learned about board leadership; and my executive director colleagues who kept me honest and helped me to universalize my own experience—Rosann Wisman, Mark Salo, Sue Momeyer, Lee Minto, Allie Stickney, and Gloria Feldt. From the regional offices in Atlanta and San Francisco, I heard from Gerry Cook, Norah Holmgren, and Bob Blomberg, whose regional jobs have given them the experience to view affiliate boards at difficult moments and during their greatest triumphs.

Several Planned Parenthood colleagues provided very helpful critiques on early drafts. I thank Allie Stickney from Portland, Oregon; Joan Babbott from Los Angeles; Debby Bergh and Mary Rauh from Northern New England; Norah Holmgren from the Western Regional office in San Francisco; Mark Salo from San Diego; and Marilyn Bowie from New York. I thank the PPFA executive staff who reacted to several chapters and to Eve Paul who reviewed the final text. To Allie Stickney goes the supreme accolade: She even reviewed and made valuable suggestions to the manuscript a second time. The stories of the Seattle and Kalamazoo affiliates' grace-under-pressure came respectively from their executive directors, Lee Minto and Louise Safron.

At my own affiliate, Planned Parenthood of Northern New England, I want to thank my board members who have proven just how possible board excellence can be, who have unflinchingly supported my work on this project, and who gave me the sabbatical leave I needed to complete it. Thanks to Brenda Adrian, Laurel Brownell, Lisa Daudon, and Rebecca Brookes, who kept the project going by supplying their talents and suggestions. Thanks to Carlie Goodrich who word processed it all through a computer conversion that played format games with the text, and saved the "almost final" version when the ceiling literally caved in, bringing with it four inches of water.

Finally, my unending gratitude goes to Karen Burke LeFevre, whose editorial skills helped immensely.

BIBLIOGRAPHY

Board Papers. San Francisco: Planned Parenthood Federation of America Western Region, 1991.

Board Responsibility. New York: Planned Parenthood Federation of America, 1991.

Cobrin, Jill. *Board Responsibility.* New York: Planned Parenthood Federation of America, 1991.

Carver, John. *Boards That Make a Difference: A New Design for Leadership in Nonprofit and Public Organizations.* San Francisco: Jossey-Bass, 1990.

Carver, John. *Consulting with Boards of Human Service Agencies: Leverage for Organizational Effectiveness.* Carmel, Indiana: Carver Governance Design, Inc., 1984.

Carver, John. *Handout Cover.* Carmel, Indiana: Carver Governance Design, Inc., no date.

Carver, John. *Redefining the Board's Role in Fiscal Planning.* Nonprofit Management and Leadership, 1991.

Cook, Jerry. *Executive Director Evaluation Guide.* Atlanta: Planned Parenthood Federation of America/Southern Region Council, 1989.

Dayton, Kenneth. *Governance is Governance.* Washington, D.C.: Independent Sector, 1987.

Drucker, Peter. *Lessons for Successful Nonprofit Governance.* In Nonprofit Management Leadership. San Francisco: Jossey-Bass Inc., 1990.

Gray, Madeline. *Margaret Sanger: A Biography of the Champion of Birth Control.* New York: Richard Marek Publishers, 1979.

Holmgren, Norah. *Board Papers.* San Francisco: Planned Parenthood Federation of America, 1992.

Holmgren, Norah. *The Board Officer's Manual.* San Francisco: Planned Parenthood Federation of America Western Region, 1990.

Hood, Paul, and Harry Jennings. *The Non-Profits Guide to Creating an Effective Governing Board.* Richmond, Virginia: Jennings, Hood and Associates, 1984.

Issues Manual. New York: Planned Parenthood Federation of America, 1986.

Johnson, Jane. *An Analysis of Executive Director Turnover in 1990.* New York: Planned Parenthood Federation of America, 1991.

Johnson, Jane. *The Mission Is the Message: The Healing Planned Parenthood Affiliate Now and in 1997.* New York: Planned Parenthood Federation of America, 1987.

Kantner, Margaret A. *Board/CEO Relationships.* Washington, D.C.: Independent Sector (from *Effective Sector Leadership Management Quarterly*), 1988.

Karn, G. Neil. *Business of Boards Is Serious Business.* Voluntary Action Leadership, 1983.

Keller, Vaughn. *Oh No, Not Another Meeting!: The Non-Profit Board of Directors.* Westport, Connecticut: The Riverside Group, 1981.

Keller, Vaughn. *Strategic Planning Handbook.* New York: Planned Parenthood Federation of America, 1983.

Lord, James Gregory. *The Raising of Money: Thirty-five Essentials Every Trustee Should Know.* Cleveland: Third Sector Press, 1983.

Minto, Lee. *Choosing An Effective Executive Director: A Guide for Affiliate Boards.* Seattle: Planned Parenthood of Seattle-King County, 1983.

Minto, Lee. *Planning for the Future: A Guide for Planned Parenthood Boards.* Seattle: Planned Parenthood of Seattle-King County, 1983.

O'Connell, Brian. *The Board Members Book: Making a Difference in Voluntary Organizations.* The Foundation Center, 79 Fifth Ave., New York, NY 10003-3050. Copyright 1985 by Brian O'Connell. Reprinted by permission.

O'Connell, Brian. *The Role of the Board and Board Members.* Washington, D.C.: Independent Sector, 1988.

Panas, Jerold. *Boardroom Verities: A Celebration of Trusteeship with Some Guides and Techniques to Govern By.* Chicago: Precept Press, Inc., 1991.

Planned Parenthood 2000: A Planning and Discussion Paper developed by the Members of MEXDICO, 1987.

PPFA Strategic Plan 1989-1993. New York: Planned Parenthood Federation of America, 1988.

PPNNE Board Policy Manual. Williston, Vermont. Planned Parenthood of Northern New England, 1986.

Salo, Mark. *A Not-for-Profit Planning Model.* San Diego: Planned Parenthood/San Diego and Riverside Counties, 1991.

Sanger, Margaret. Quotations are from Madeline Gray, *Margaret Sanger.* Noted above.

Saunier, Anne. *Organizing Volunteers to Get Results.* New York: Planned Parenthood Federation of America, 1989.

Schleck, Roth. *Building a Quality Board.* Madison, Wisconsin: Nonprofit World, 1985.

Swanson, Andrew. *Building a Better Board.* Washington, D.C.: Taft Corporation, 1984.

Swanson, Andrew. *Evaluation—Bane? or Boon?* Rushford, Rhode Island: Community Services Consultants, Ltd., 1980.

Tepper, Sheri. *On Being Board: How Not to be Deadwood.* Lakewood, Colorado: RAJ Publications, 1986.